EXERCISE THERAPY

Dr. Suraj Kumar

SHREE PUBLISHERS & DISTRIBUTORS
New Delhi–110 002

Edition : 2009
Revised Edition : 2018

Published by :
SHREE PUBLISHERS & DISTRIBUTORS
22/4735 Prakash Deep Building,
Ansari Road, Darya Ganj,
New Delhi–110 002

ISBN : 978–81–8329–317–4

Printed by :
Delhi Printer & Lamination
New Delhi–110 002

Dedicated

to

My Beloved

Father & Mother

Sh. Rajkumar Sinha

&

Smt. Manorama Sinha

FOREWORD

It is always a pleasure to be asked to write a foreword to a Book of Exercise Therapy when you admire the author and approve its contents. This book along with different chapters of various subjects of Exercise Therapy inclusive of Hydrotherapy, Gait, Muscle Testing, Gymnasium, Mat Exercise and Therapeutic Exercises which is knowledgable for students as well as practicing physiotherapists.

The author, Suraj Kumar is the best teacher, an innovator and a person with a quick and receptive brain, always willing to learn himself and modify his approach and teaching in the light of wide experience.

I have been lucky enough to work with him and I think it is important for his profession to retain the name of the original author of a valuable book. I hope that this book will continue for many years to stimulate students in learning.

Prof. V.P. Sharma

M.S. (Ortho), D.N.B. (PMR), P.G. Spine (Aust.)

FACS, FICS, FIMSA, MAMS

Director–Professor & Head

Deptt. of Physical Medicine Rehabilitation

C.S.M. Medical University, Lucknow-18

(Upgraded K.G. Medical University)

PREFACE

There is no permanent cure by medicine for chronic diseases like Cervical pain, Backache, Arthritis etc. One can only take some medicines and pain killers to subside his pain temporarily. This is because this type of treatment only provide symptomatic relief and doesn't remove the root cause of the problem. Exercise comes to rescue at such moments and can provide permanent relief if one has patience to pursue it regularly with interest. By maintaining good postures, derived postures, mobilization, relaxation, loosening and strengthening exercises for muscles, one can restore the muscles and spine in their proper tone and alignment provided they have not undergone degenerative and irreversible structural changes. In this book I have tried to explain scientifically various aspects related to therapeutic exercises, principles of exercises and physics behind the exercises so that general readers/students and apologize for any mistake if left out inadvertently.

Many friends have helped me along the path of exercises to the place where I can share something of what I know in this book. I am grateful to all of them; but especially want to acknowledge & thank those who have taught me: Dr. Manda Chauhan, Dr. Rajni Kalra, Dr. Chandan Chawla, Dr. Tripta Gahi, Dr. D. Vijay Kumar, Dr. A.K. Jain, Dr. V.P. Sharma and H.K. Tripathi. I am grateful to my students for giving me the opportunity and privilege to teaching and for showing me that this book was needed. Among them, special thanks are due to P.D. Tiwar, Mahesh Tiwari, Lal Bahudur, Vishal, Amit Kumar and Miraj for believing in the book and for editing it.

Special thanks to Rahul R. Verma, Rajeeb Lochan Das for lovely drawings that enhanced the book's appeal and usefulness, and finally I am grateful to them for contribution.

Dr. Suraj Kumar

Contents

1

INTRODUCTION

PHYSIOTHERAPY

Physiotherapy is a branch of medical science which deals the patients with the help of physical modalities (heat, hydrotherapy, cold, current etc) and different types of exercises.

According to Delhi Council of Physiotherapy: "Physiotherapy means physiotherapeutic system of medicine which includes examination, treatment, advice and instructions to any person preparatory to or for the purpose of or in connection with movement dysfunction, body malfunction, physical disorder, disability, healing and pain from trauma and disease, physical and mental conditions using physical agents including exercise, mobilization, manipulation, mechanical and electrotherapy, activity and devices or diagnosis, treatment and prevention".

According to Maharashtra Council of Physiotherapy: "Physiotherapy means a branch of modern medical science which includes examination, assessment, interpretation, physical diagnosis, planning and execution of treatment and advice to any person for the purpose of preventing, correcting, alleviating and limiting dysfunction, acute and chronic body malfunction including life saving measures via chest physiotherapy in the intensive care units, curing physical disorders or disability promoting physical fitness, facilitating healing and pain relief and treatment of physical and psychosomatic disorders through modulating physiological and physical response using physical agent, activities and devices using exercises, mobilization manipulations, therapeutic ultra-sound, electrical ar agents and electrotherapy for diagnosis, treatr prevention".

PHYSIOTHERAPIST

Physiotherapist is able to prevent, identify, assess, correct or evaluate the acute or prolong movement disorders.

Or

Physiotherapists analyze the impact of injury, disease or disorders on movements and functions. Their unique contribution to health care is to promote, restore and prolong physical independence by enhancing a client's functional capacity. Physiotherapists encourage clients to assume responsibility for their health and participate in team approaches to health service delivery.

PHYSIOTHERAPY INCLUDES

Assessing the Patient

Planning and implementing the programme after assessment.

Altering and continuing management programme after reassessment.

- Assessment of clients with actual or potential impairments, pain, functional limitations, disabilities or other health-related conditions using detailed history-taking, as well as specific tests and measures for screening, establishing a diagnosis and monitoring.
- Diagnosis resulting from assessment findings and clinical reasoning to determine abilities, functional needs and potential for change.
- Planning an intervention strategy that addresses the prognosis and follow-up and incorporates the application of selected approaches and techniques supported by the best evidence available.
- Implementing selected interventions safely to relieve pain; achieve and maintain health and fitness, functional independence and physical performance and manage the identified impairments, disabilities and limits to participation.

- Evaluation of health status as a baseline for monitoring or to determine the result, impact, or effectiveness of physiotherapy intervention,
- Education of the profession, other health professionals, the public and clients with the intention of transferring knowledge and skills and developing understanding, independence and competence.
- Consultation that provides professional advice and solutions addressing a wide range of health service and health status issues.
- Research that encompasses the application of critical inquiry, as well as participation in or assessment of findings from research activities.
- Service management related to planning, directing, organizing and monitoring service delivery and effective utilization of resources.
- Communication with clients, team members and others to achieve collaboration and service coordination.

OBJECTIVES OF PHYSIOTHERAPY

Physiotherapy is a health profession that deals with management of body dysfunction or disorder by physical modalities. The aims of physiotherapeutic system are to promote option at human health and function through the application of medical health sciences and clinical sciences. Physiotherapy is a first contact, autonomous, client-focused health profession which dedicated to following objectives:

- Improving and maintaining functional independence and physical performance.
- Preventing and managing pain, physical impairments, disabilities and limits to participation.
- Promoting fitness, health and wellness.

AIMS OF PHYSIOTHERAPY

Physiotherapy used in restoration of ph
and maintenance of physical well being are the

therapy. The physiotherapy is works for the coordinal principle of rehabilitation science i.e. to treat the patient as a whole person. Following points are the major aims of physiotherapy:-

- Relieving and treating pains
- Maintaining or improving of mobility of joints
- Maintaining and increasing the strength of muscles
- Re-educating muscles
- Correction of posture
- Preventing contracture and deformity
- Increasing vital capacity to maintain general body function
- Healing of wound and ulcer etc
- Maintain and improving co-ordination
- To give advice related to waste and physical work
- Suggestion for general health of the body
- Facilitating motor function
- Facilitating normal development

SCOPE OF PHYSIOTHERAPY

Physiotherapy has a wide scope. Physiotherapist may join following organization:-

- Government job
- Sports
- Teaching
- N.G.O. (Non governmental organization)
- Hospital
- Nursing home
- Hospices
- Special school
- Rehabilitation centre
- Health and Fitness centre or Gymnasium
- Private clinic
- Maternity clinic
- Research centre
- Foreign countries

DIMENSION OF PHYSIOTHERAPY

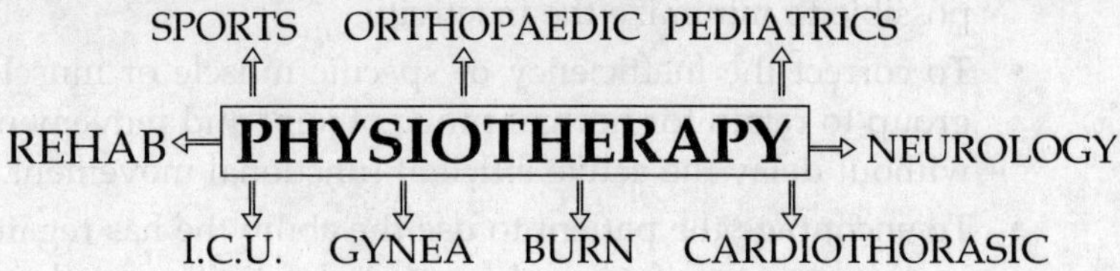

Fig. 1.1: *Dimension of Physiotherapy*

Pediatrics	Cerebral palsy (C.P.), Developmental delay, Spina bifida.
Orthopedic	Musculoskeletal disorder as back pain, knee pain, cervical pain, arthritis, fracture and other spinal deformities.
Cardiothoracic	Lungs congestion, Thoracic surgeries, Asthma, Bronchitis, Lung abscess, Pneumonia.
Neurology	Hemiplegia, Quadriplegia, Paraplegia, Bell's palsy.
I.C.U.	Management for chronic and emergency condition of patient.
Rehabilitation Center	The centre which helps for disabled person. e.g. – Contracture, Deformity, Amputation, Shortening of limbs.
Sports	Sports injury, Sprain, Muscle fatigue, Strain, Ligament pull.
	(R – Rest, I – Ice, C – Compression, E – Elevation)
Gynaecology	Back care after delivery, Prolapsed uterus, Pre and post natal exercises.
Burn	Contracture of muscle, Keloids, Scar.

BRANCHES OF PHYSIOTHERAPY

1. Exercise therapy
2. Electrotherapy

Exercise Therapy

Aims of exercise therapy:

- To promote the activity whenever and wherever it is possible to minimize the inactivity.
- To correct the inefficiency of specific muscle or muscle group to retain for normal range of joint and movement without delay the active efficient functional movement.
- To encourage the patient to use the ability he has regain in performance of normal functional activity and show accelerates the rehabilitation.

Electrotherapy

Aims of electrotherapy:

- To promote normal physiological process by application of electrical stimulus to body parts.
- To enhance the cellular metabolic activity by entering waves / rays inside the body.
- To provide heating and cooling effect according to the requirement in various dysfunction.

OO

2

MECHANICAL PRINCIPLE FOR EXERCISE THERAPY

AXIS

Axis is an imaginary line around which movement takes place for any object.

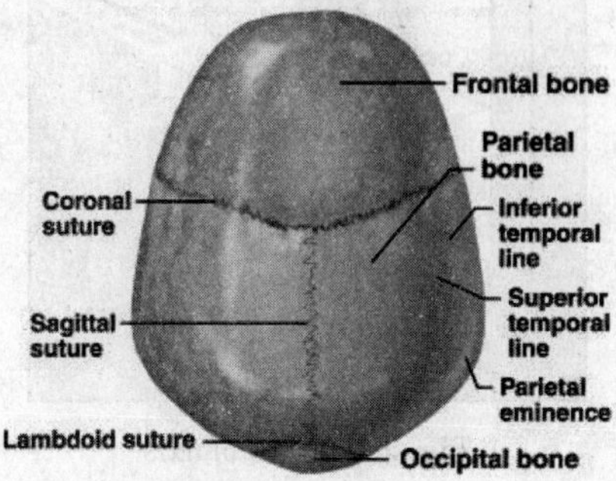

Types of Axis

Coronal axis / Medio-lateral axis

Coronal axis is parallel to the coronal suture of skull, movement about this axis is in sagital plane eg. forward & backward motion such as flexion & extension of lumbar. (Fig. 2.1 A)

Sagital axis or Anterior – Posterior axis

Sagital axis is parallel to the sagital suture of skull i.e. Anteroposterior in direction, Movement about this axis is in frontal plane. (Fig. 2.1 B).

Vertical axis or Longitudinal axis

It is parallel to the line of gravity. Movement about this axis is in horizontal (Transverse) plane (Fig. 2.1 C).

All flexion and extension movement in the body, are always takes place in frontal axis and sagital plane. In fundamental standing position the centre of gravity lies in body of the second sacral vertebrae.

All adduction and abduction movement takes place in sagital axis and frontal plane. All rotation movement inside the body takes place in vertical axis and transverse plane.

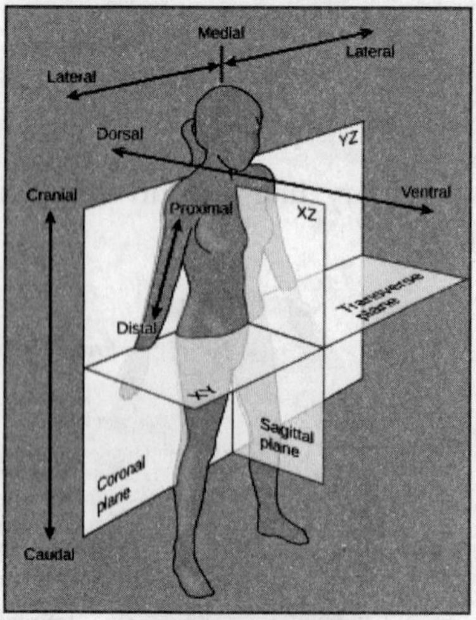

Fig. 2.1: *Types of axis*

PLANE

Plane is an imaginary surface through which movement takes place. Axis and plane are always perpendicular to each other.

Types of Plane

Transverse / Horizontal plane

X coordinates divided the body into two parts i.e. upper half and lower half. X coordinate corresponds to transverse plane (Horizontal plane). (Fig. 2.2).

Frontal plane / Coronal plane

Y coordinate divided the body into anterior half and posterior half. Y coordinate corresponds to frontal (Coronal) plane. (Fig. 2.2).

Sagital plane

Z coordinate divides the body in to two parts i.e. right and left. Z coordinate corresponds to sagital plane. (Fig. 2.2).

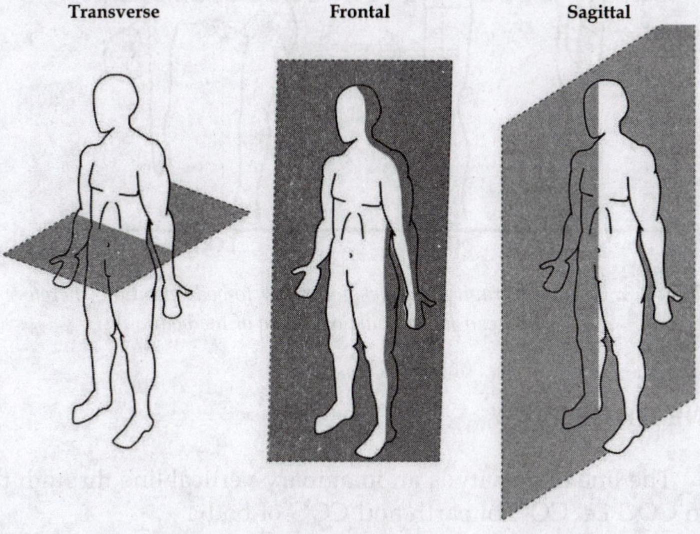

Fig. 2.2: *The plane: X–Transverse / Horizontal plane, Y–Forntal / Coronal plane, Z–Sagital plane.*

CENTER OF GRAVITY (COG)

Center of gravity is an imaginary point where whole mass of body is concentrated.

In human body COG is situated anterior to the second sacral vertebrae. This position is applied only in the anatomical standing position.

Location of centre of gravity is depend not only arrangement of body segment but also depend on the mass of the body (Distribution of mass and also shape of the object). (Fig. 2.3). COG can falls outside or inside of the body.

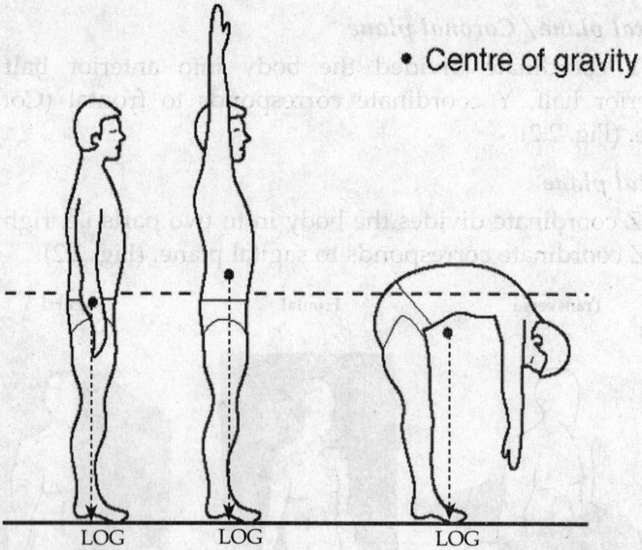

Fig. 2.3: *Centre of gravity changes according to body position, therefore COG can fall outside or inside of the body*

LINE OF GRAVITY

The line of gravity is an imaginary vertical line through the two COG i.e. COG of earth and COG of body.

In human body the line of gravity passes through the anterior to the second sacral vertebrae, the vertex and the point between the feet, level with the transverse tarsal joint in the anatomical standing position.

BASE OF SUPPORT

Base of support is the area by which human body is supported. (Fig. 2.4). For an object the line of gravity must fall within the base of support, the object must be stable. When the line of gravity falls outside the base of support with object will tend to fall. Larger the base of support of an object, greater the stability of that object. Closer the centre of gravity to the base of support, provide maximum stability.

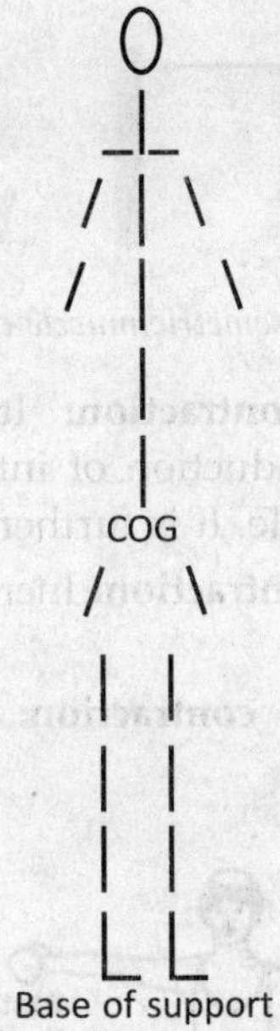

Fig. 2.4: *Base of support*

MUSCLE CONTRACTION

Muscle contraction is a production of intramuscular tension with or without change in the length of muscle.

Types of Muscle Contractions

There are two types of muscle contractions according to the length of muscle while contracting of muscle occurs-

1. Isometric Muscle contraction
2. Isotonic Muscle contraction

Isometric Muscle contraction: It is a type of muscle contraction in which production of intramuscular tension without change in length of muscle. Work done is equal to zero. (Fig. 2.5, 2.6. B)

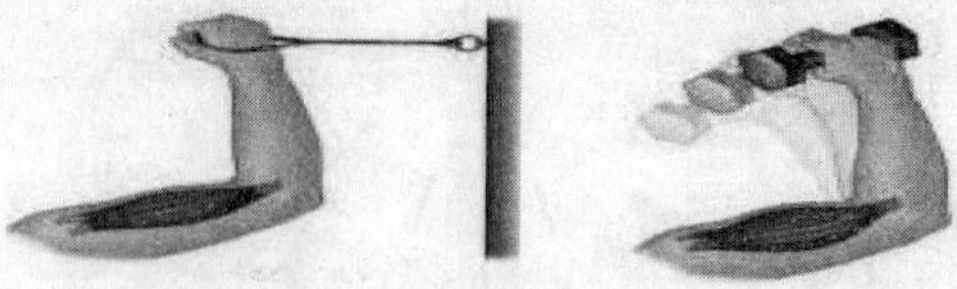

Fig. 2.5: *Isometric muscle contraction*

Isotonic Muscle contraction: It is a type of muscle contraction in which production of intramuscular tension with change in length of muscle. It is further divided into two types -

Eccentric muscle contraction: Increase in length of muscle. (Fig. 2.6A).

Concentric muscle contraction: Decrease in length of muscle. (Fig. 2.6C).

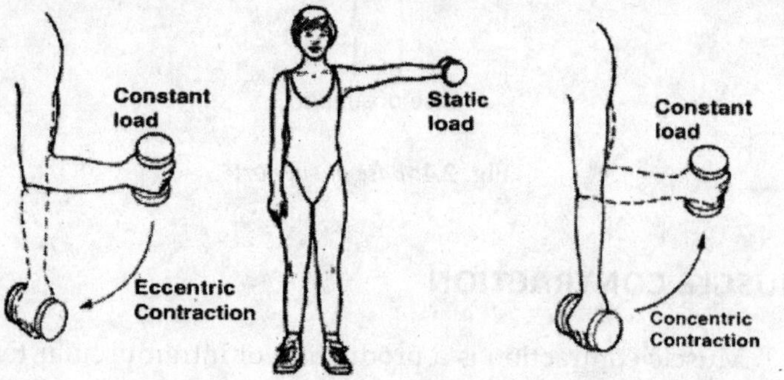

A–Eccentric contraction, B–Isometric conctrection, C–Concentric contraction

Fig. 2.6: *Muscle contraction*

Muscular Work

It is a multiplication of force generated by the muscle and change in length of muscle. Muscles work involves as in intramuscular tension. It is of three types:

1. *Static muscle work*

Work done by isometric contraction is zero, because of no displacement and some amount of force generated by muscles, so the muscle work is zero. As for example- Suppose force generated by Biceps muscle is 40 Newton and displacement is 0, then-

Muscle work by biceps = F × D

= 40 × 0

= 0

2. *Concentric muscle work*

In this condition some amount of force generated by the muscle and there is decrease in length of muscle by contract isotonic contraction. In this case force generated by muscle resists the external force applied on it, resulting in maximum work.

3. *Eccentric muscle work*

In this condition the muscle contract isotonically to increase in the length of muscle. External force is more than internal force, resulting in minimum work.

Range of the Muscle Work

The range of muscle work is the extent of muscular contraction which results in joint movement. (Fig. 2.7).

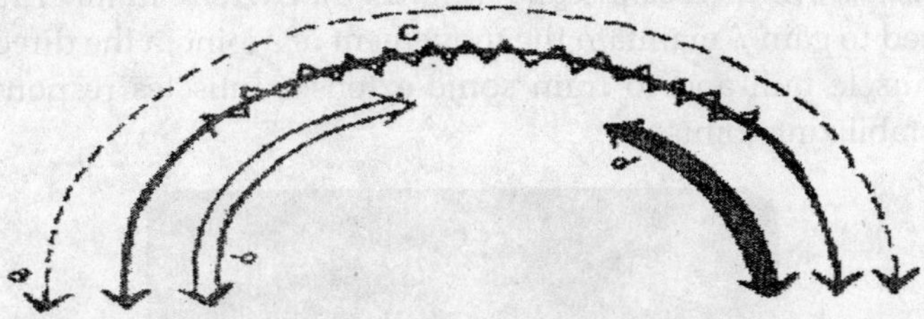

Position of full contraction **Position of full stretch**

a = Full Range, b = Inner Range, c = Middle Range, d = Outer Range

Fig. 2.7: *Range of the muscle work*

Full Range

The joint is moved as the muscle work from the position in which they are fully stretched, to the position in which they are fully contracted concentrically or from the position of full contraction to the position of maximum stretch, if they are working eccentrically. (Fig. 2.7A).

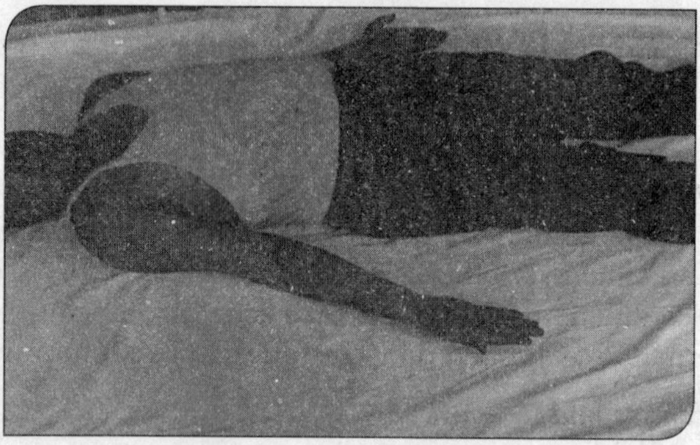

Fig. 2.7A: *Full range of the muscle work*

Inner Range

The muscle work either concentrically from position in which it is partially contracted (approximately halfway between the limit of full range) to a position of full contraction, or vice versa, if it works eccentrically. (Fig. 2.7B). Exercise in inner range is used to gain / maintain the movement of a joint in the direction of muscle pull and to train some extensor muscles responsible for stabilizing joints.

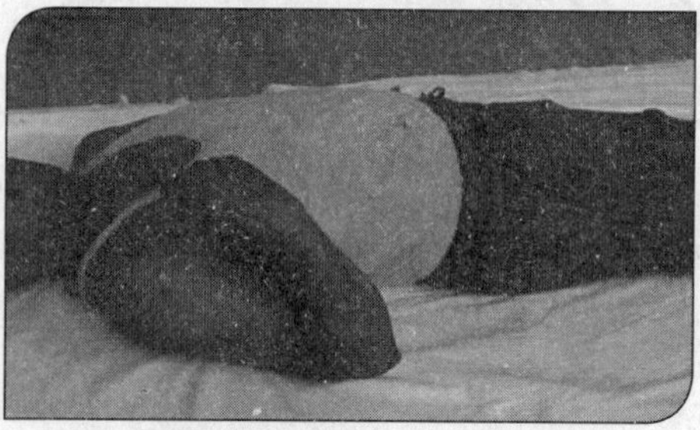

Fig. 2.7B: *Inner range of the muscle work*

Outer Range

Muscle work concentrically forms the position in which they are fully stretched to a position in which they are partially (half) contracted or vice versa if working eccentrically. (Fig. 2.7C). The outer range of muscle work is used extensively in muscle reeducation as a contraction is initiated more easily from stretch in most muscle.

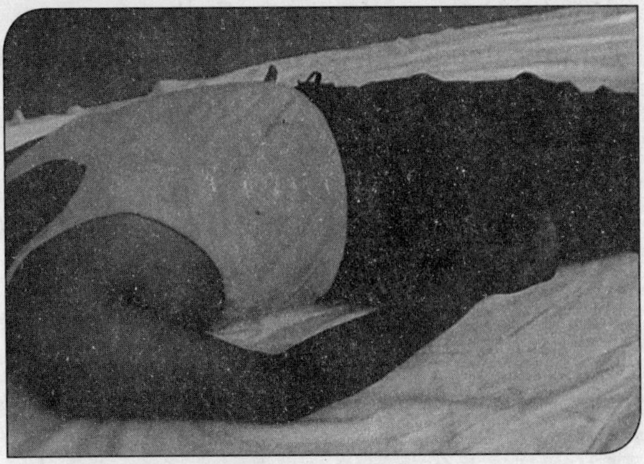

Fig. 2.7C: *Outer range of the muscle work*

Middle Range

Muscle work in the form of partially contracted and partially stretched position of muscle. (Fig. 2.7D).

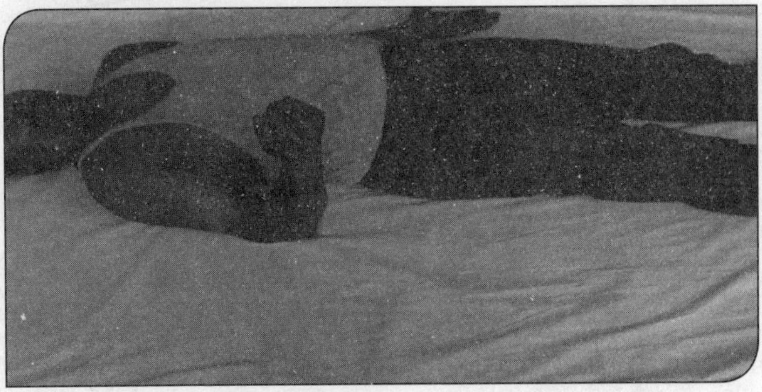

Fig. 2.7D: *Middle range of the muscle work*

LEVER

Lever is a rigid bar which is capable of movement about a fix point which is called fulcrum.

1. Work is done when a force or effort (E) is applied at one point (F) on the lever act upon another force or weight (W) along at second point on the lever.
2. For preparation of lever there are 3 points as follows:

   E = efforts

   F = Fulcrum

   W = weight
3. Effort arm - It is perpendicular distance from fulcrum to effort is known as effort arm. It is denoted as EA. (Fig. 2.8).

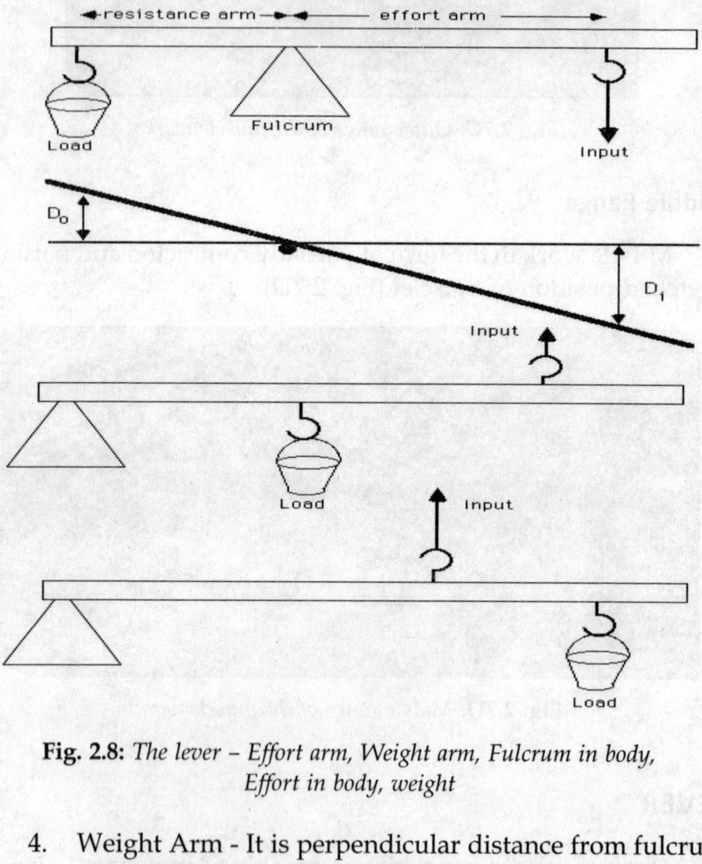

Fig. 2.8: *The lever – Effort arm, Weight arm, Fulcrum in body, Effort in body, weight*

4. Weight Arm - It is perpendicular distance from fulcrum to weight is known as weight arm or resistant arm. It is denoted as WA. (Fig. 2.8).

5. Fulcrum in body - In human body lever is represent by bone which is capable of movement at a fix point known as fulcrum, formed at articulating surface or joint. (Fig. 2.8).
6. Effort in body - Effort which works the lever is supplied by force of muscle contraction applied at the point of insertion to the bone. (Fig. 2.8).
7. Weight - It may be either center of gravity or the part move object to be lifted. (Fig. 2.8).

Classification of Lever

In human body there are 3 orders of lever. Each lever characterized by the position of fulcrum, weight and effort-

1st order lever (Fig. 2.9A).

2nd order lever (Fig. 2.9B).

3rd order lever (Fig. 2.9C).

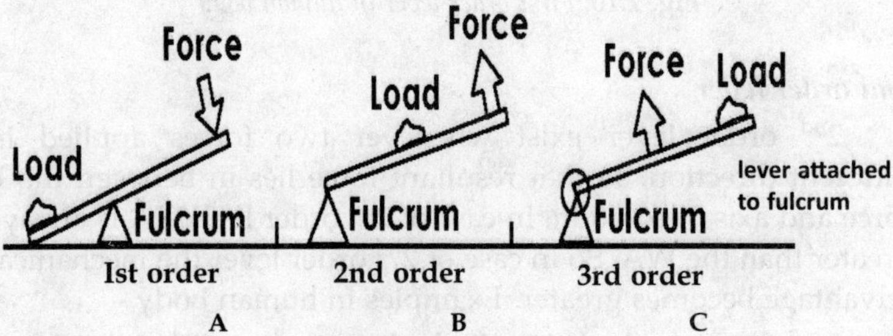

Fig. 2.9: *Classification of lever*

1st order lever

1st order lever system exists whenever two resultant forces are applied on either side of axis at some distance from that axis creating rotation in opposite direction. In 1st order lever system effort arm may be greater than weight arm or smaller than weight arm or similar than weight arm. Examples in human body –

During nodding movements of the head, the skull represents the lever, the Atlanto-occipital joints act as a fulcrum, the weight is situated anteriorly in the face, and the effort is supplied by the contraction of posterior neck muscle. (Fig. 2.10).

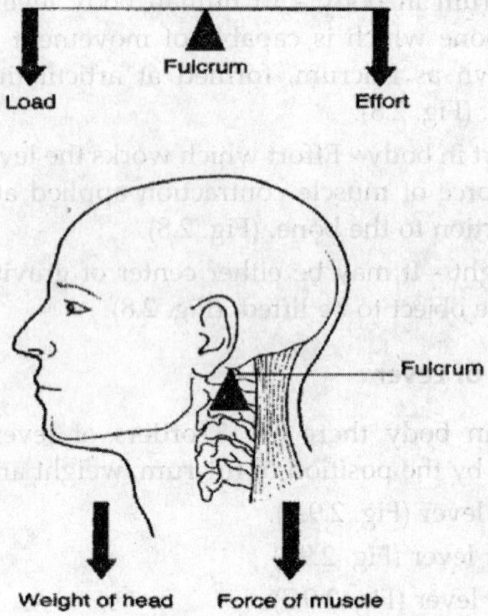

Fig. 2.10: *First order lever in human body*

2nd order lever

2nd order lever exist whenever two forces applied in different direction, so that resultant force lies in between the E force and axis of rotation. In case of 2nd order lever EA is always greater than the WA. So in case of 2nd order lever the mechanical advantage becomes greater. Examples in human body –

In human body lower limb demonstrate 2nd order lever when heel raised to stand on toes. Tarsal and metatarsal bone are established by muscular action to form lever, the fulcrum is on metatarsol-phalangeal joint and weight is transmitted through the talus bone, and the effort is applied on insertion point of Tendocalcaneus by contraction of calf muscle. In the arm the action of brachioradialis muscle in flexing the elbow joint can be taken as another example (Fig. 2.11).

3rd order lever

It exists whenever the force of lever is applied so that the effort force lies close to the fulcrum of lever. In case of 3rd order lever the WA is always greater than EA. In case of 3rd order lever the Machenical Advantages (MA) is always less than 1. The loss of MA is weighted by the advantage gained by speed, ROM. Examples in human body:

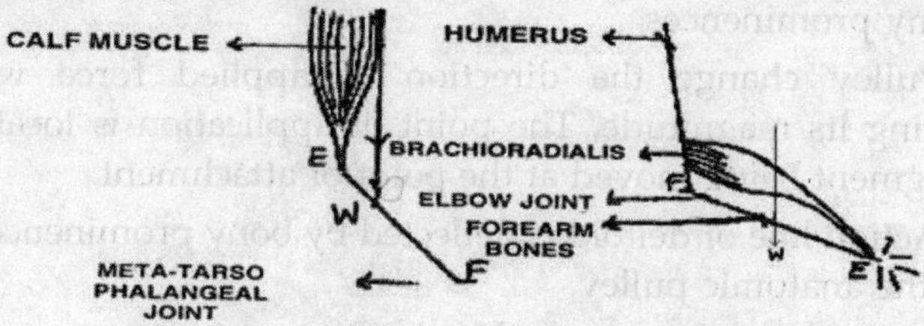

Fig. 2.11: *Second order lever in human body.*

When the forearm act as a lever and fulcrum at elbow joint, effort is produced by the biceps muscle at the point of radial tuberosity and weight is provided by the hand and forearm. Another example, in prone lying position flexion at the knee joint performed by hamstring muscle. In this case tibia acts as a lever, fulcrum at the knee joint, effort at insertion point of hamstring muscle i.e. upper posterior part of tibia and weight by the foot and lower leg. (Fig. 2.12)

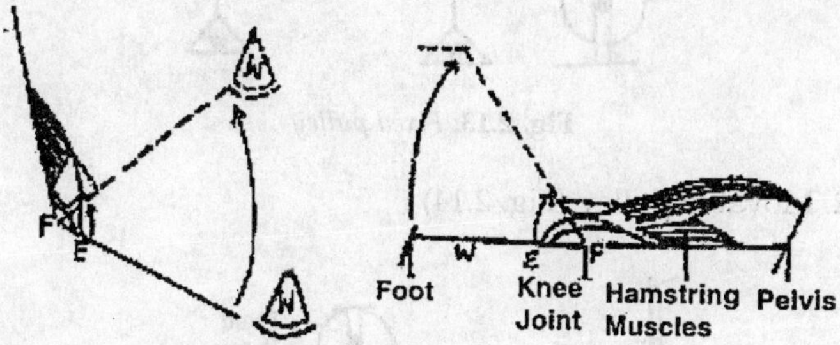

Fig. 2.12: *Third order lever in human body.*

MA of 2nd order lever > MA of 3rd order lever

In 1st order lever MA ><= 1

In 2nd order lever MA > 1

In 3rd order lever MA < 1

This type of lever is always lesser than 2nd order lever.

PULLEY

Pulley is grooved wheel which is rotated about a fixed axis by a rope which is passes around it. In human body the fibres of muscle and muscle tendon wrap around a bone or are deflected by bony prominences.

Pulley change the direction of applied force without changing its magnitude. The point of application is located on the segment being moved at the point of attachment.

Action line of deltoid is deflected by bony prominences that form the anatomic pulley.

Action line is the direction of pull that the fibres of tendon of muscle create at the point of application.

Types of Pulley

There are two types of pulley:

1. Fixed pulley (Fig. 2.13)

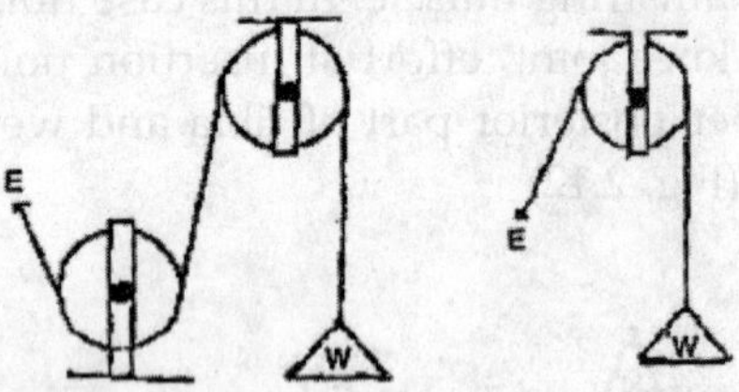

Fig. 2.13: *Fixed pulley*

2. Movable pulley (Fig. 2.14)

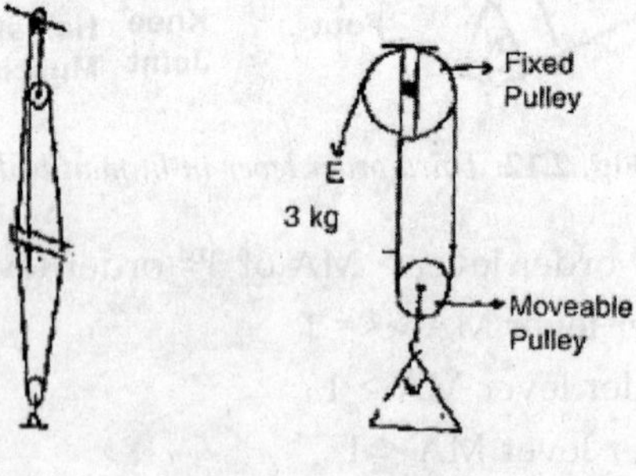

Fig. 2.14: *Movable pulley*

Arrangements of Pulleys

Single Fixed. (Fig. 2.15 a).
Single Movable. (Fig. 2.15 b).
Single Fixed & Single Movable. (Fig. 2.15 c).
Double Fixed & Single Movable. (Fig. 2.15 d).
Double Fixed & Double Movable. (Fig. 2.15 e).

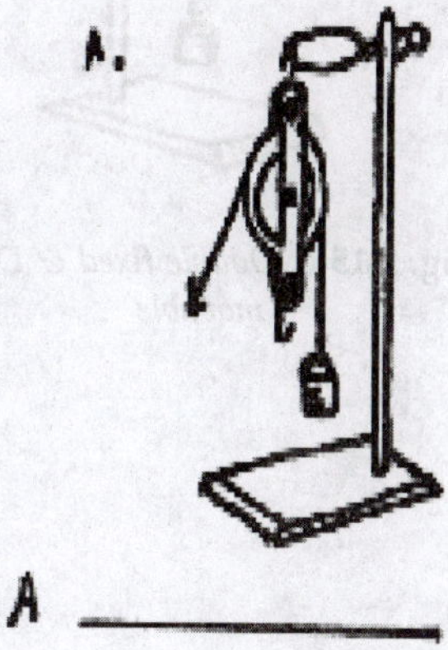

Fig. 2.15 a: *Single fixed pulley*

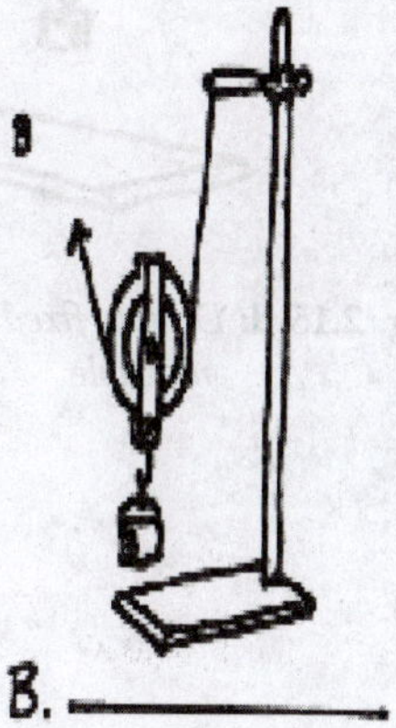

Fig. 2.15 b: *Single movable*

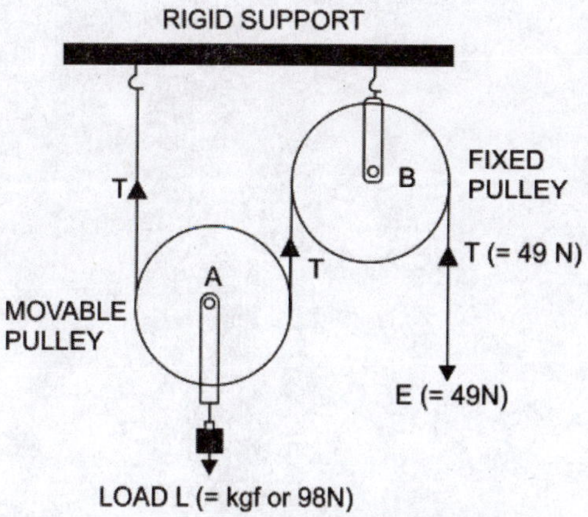

Fig. 2.15 c: *Single fixed & Single movable*

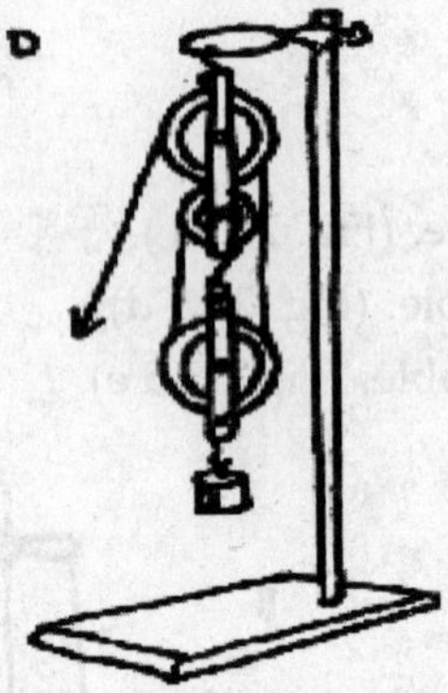

Fig. 2.15 d: *Double fixed & Single movable*

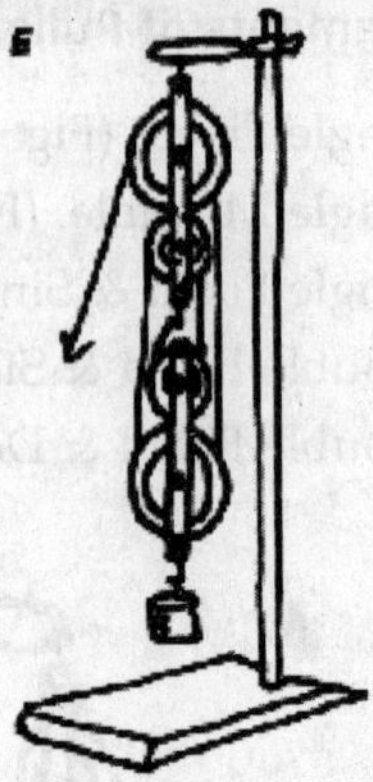

Fig. 2.15 e: *Double fixed & Double movable*

3

POSTURE

INTRODUCTION

Posture is an attitude assumed by the body either with support or without support during muscular activity or by coordination of many muscles working to maintain stability.

TYPE OF POSTURE

1. Active (walking, running, swimming)
2. Inactive (Sitting, Lying, Standing)

Active Posture

Most Muscle work is required to maintain body function and stability. It is further divided into 2 types:

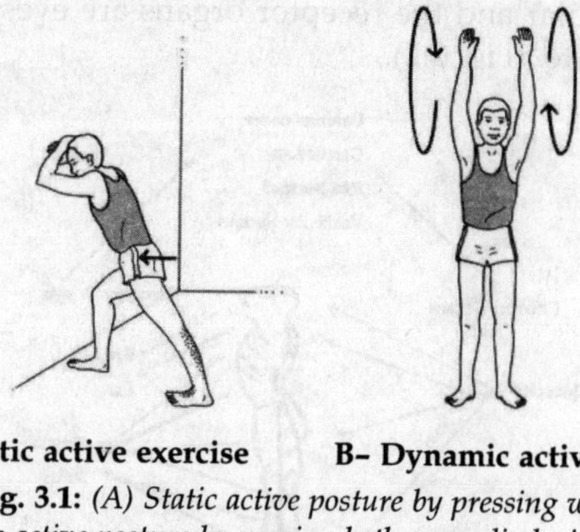

A–Static active exercise **B– Dynamic active exercise**

Fig. 3.1: *(A) Static active posture by pressing wall, (B) Dynamic active posture by moving both upper limbs in a circle form*

Static active posture—Standing, Hanging, Kneeling, Pressing wall (Fig. 3.1 A).

Dynamic active posture—Walking, moving both upper limb in a circle form, Running. (Fig. 3.1 B)

Inactive or passive or resting posture or sleeping posture

There is minimum demand upon the muscle that is responsible for the maintenance for essential body function.

POSTURAL CONTROL

Person's ability to maintain stability of the body and body segments is known as posture control.

Static posture controls involves maintenance of the particulars posture against gravity while dynamic posture control maintenance of stability during movement of body or body segment.

Control of posture depends upon the integrity of the visual system, musculoskeletal system, vestibular system etc.

CNS must capable of revising and processing information from all system and must be able to collect information from the receptors.

Through the reflexes (reflex is an arch through the spinal cord of efferent response to an afferent stimulus).

Organ concerned with CNS are the cerebral cortex, cerebellum, red nucleus, vestibular nucleus etc. The effectors organ is muscular and the receptor organs are eyes, ears, joints, skin, muscles etc. (Fig. 3.2).

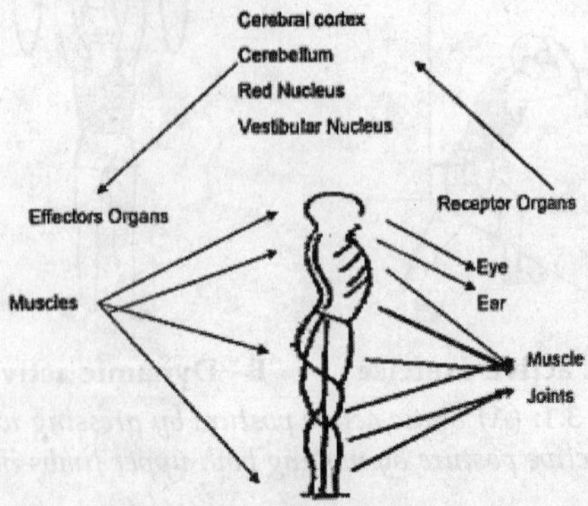

Fig. 3.2: *Postural control*

PATTERN OF POSTURE

1. Good Posture 2. Bad Posture

Good Posture

Posture is said to be good it is fulfill the purpose for which it is used with maximum efficiency and minimum effort (Fig, 3.3).

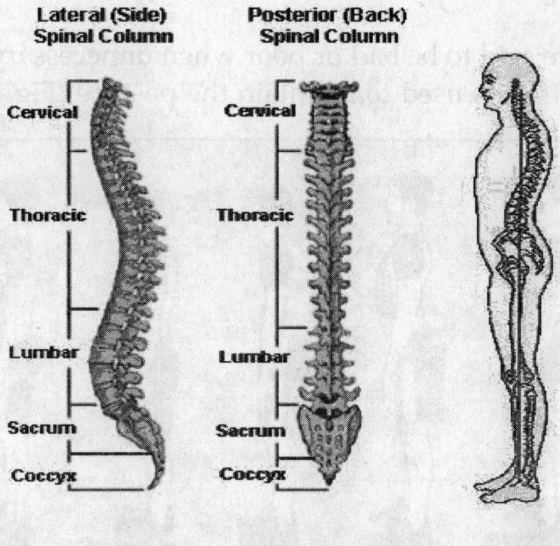

Fig, 3.3: *Spinal alignment of good posture*

For a good posture the line of gravity should pass via specific body landmarks. Any deviation can be observed in lateral view.

Line of Gravity Pass	*Body Segment*
Anterior	Atlantooccipital joint
Posterior	Cervical region
Anterior	Thoracic region
Posterior	Lumber region
Anterior	Sacroiliac joint (SI joint)
Posterior	Hip Joint
Anterior	Knee Joint
Posterior	Patella
Anterior	Ankle Joint

Development of Good Posture

- Strong Psychological background
- Good hygienic conditions
- Opportunity for plenty of natural free movement
- Healthy diet
- Height of the person

Bad Posture

Posture said to be bad or poor when unnecessary amount of muscular effort is used to maintain the posture (Fig. 3..4).

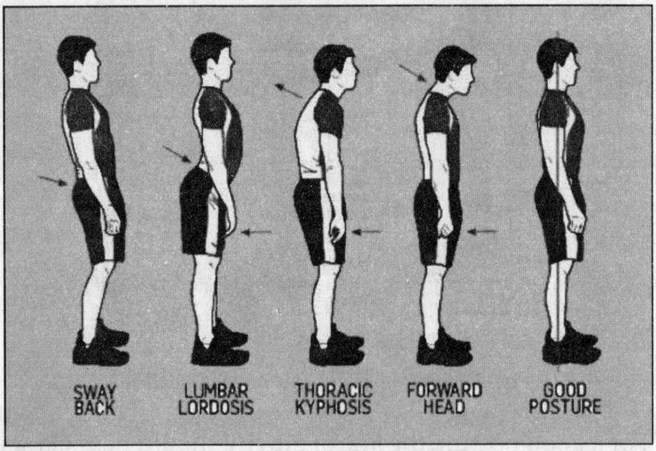

Fig. 3.4: *Bad posture*

Factors responsible for bad posture are:

- Mental attitude
- Poor hygienic condition
- Local condition (pain, muscular, weakness, muscular spasm, muscular, cramp, spasticity)
- Occupational tension

Note: A mirror, Posture recorders, Photographs, external stimulus, Bio feedback may use for postural correction & regaining good alignment.

4

FUNDAMENTAL STARTING POSITION

INTRODUCTION

Every posture follow movement like a shadow. Movement begins with posture and ends with posture. The posture from which movement is initiated is known as fundamental starting position. They may be active and passive in nature.

There are 5 fundamental positions of human body, are:

1. Standing
2. Sitting
3. Lying
4. Kneeing
5. Hanging

STANDING POSITION

Objectives

This is most difficult fundamental position to maintain as the whole body must be balanced and stabilizes in correct alignment on a small base by the co-ordinate work of many muscle groups.

Rules

- The heel are together and on the same line. The toes are slightly apart (< 45º).
- Knees are together and straight.
- The hip are extended and slightly laterally rotated.

- The pelvis is balanced on the femoral head.
- Spine is straightened to his or her maximum length.
- The vertex is thrust upward the ears are in same level and the eyes looks forwarded.
- Shoulders are in same level and back and downward.
- The arms are loose and palm facing inward towards the body.

Muscle work

- Intrinsic Muscle of foot working to stabilize feet and to prevent curling of toes so that flexes of the interphalengial joint can press the base of toes to the ground. (Fig. 4.1).

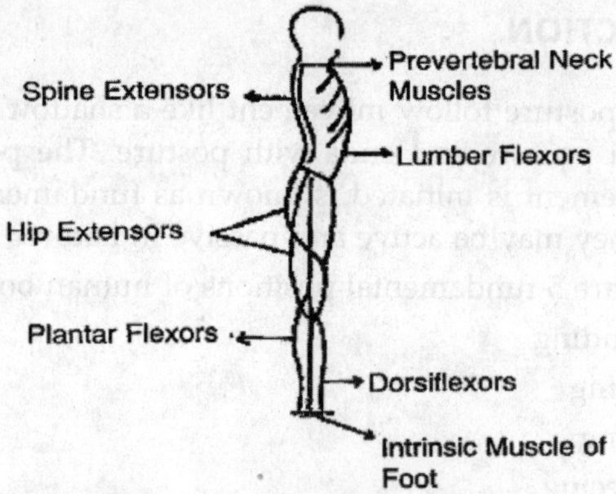

Fig. 4.1: *Muscle work in standing position*

- Dorsiflexors of the foot working to the counter the action of plantar flexors and to support the medial longitudinal arch of the foot.
- The Plantar flexors of the ankle working to balance the lower leg on the ground.
- Evertors working to counter balance of the invertors.
- The extensors of the knee i.e. quadriceps are working to keep the knee extended.
- The extensors of the hips are working to maintain hip extension and balanced to pelvis on femoral head, lateral rotator of the hip are slightly working to laterally rotate hip.

- Abdominal muscle are working to prevent over action of the extensors of this region. It also maintains the correct angle of pelvic tilt.
- Extensors of the trunk are working to keep straight the back straight.
- Prevertebral neck muscle working to control excessive extension of the neck and to straighten the cervical spine.
- Retractor of the scapula working to draw scapula backward so that the glenoid cavity faces more or less laterally.
- The arms are relaxed.
- **Effect and Uses**
- Antigravity muscle of trunk and lower limb working isometrically to hold the position.
- As the base is relatively small and C.O.G. high. The state of equilibrium of body is relatively less stable than the other fundamentals position.
- Standing is only starting position for exercise for those which is maintaining it correctly.
- The erect position of the whole body is the position of alertness on which the thorax is free and abdominal viscera are well supported. It is associated with feeling of joy and efficacy.

SITTING POSITION

Objectives

This is most difficult fundamental position to maintain as the whole body must be balanced and stabilizes in correct alignment on a small base by the co-ordinate work of many muscle groups. (Fig. 4.2).

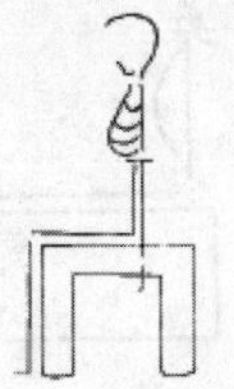

Fig. 4.2: *Fundamental sitting position*

Rules

- Hips and knee to be flexed to a right angle.
- Knees slightly apart so that both femur bone should be parallel.
- Feet must on the ground with the heel vertically below the knee.
- Rests are similar as standing position.

Muscle Work

- No muscle work of leg because legs are fully supported on chair and ground.
- Flexors of hip work to maintain right angle at hip joint.
- Rest muscles are working same as standing

Effects and Uses

- Sitting is a comfortable and very stable position which is much used and it is used particularly for those who lack strength and control to maintain a difficult position.
- It is also used in non-weight bearing exercise at knee and ankle.

KNEELING POSITION

Objectives

The body is supported on the knee which may be together or slightly apart. (Fig. 4.3).

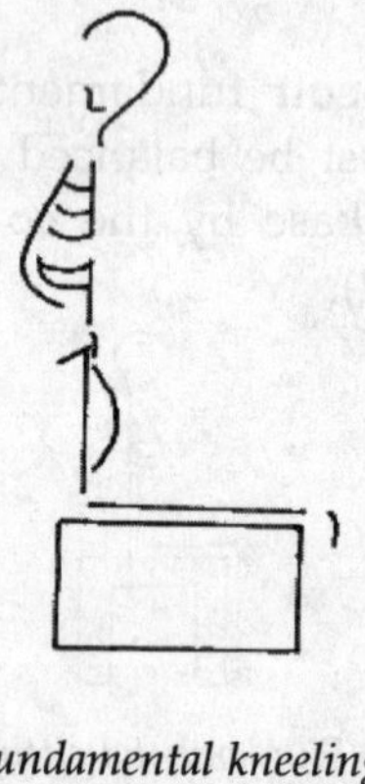

Fig. 4.3: *Fundamental kneeling position*

Rules

- Lower leg rest on the floor with the feet planter flexed or if the plinth is used the feet may be in the neutral position at the edge of plinth.
- The rest of the body held of standing position.

Muscle work

- Lower leg is relaxed. Body must be stabilizes on the knee.
- Knee flexor and extensors are working to balance vertically on the knee.
- The extensor of hip and flexor of lumbar spine works more strongly to maintain the correct angle of pelvic tilt.

Effect and uses

Although the COG of the body is relatively lower than in standing, the position is strongly more stable and uncomfortable for most of the people.

LYING POSITION

Rules and Objectives

- This is easiest fundamental position. (Fig.4.4).
- Body should be completely supported in the supine position and as stable as possible.

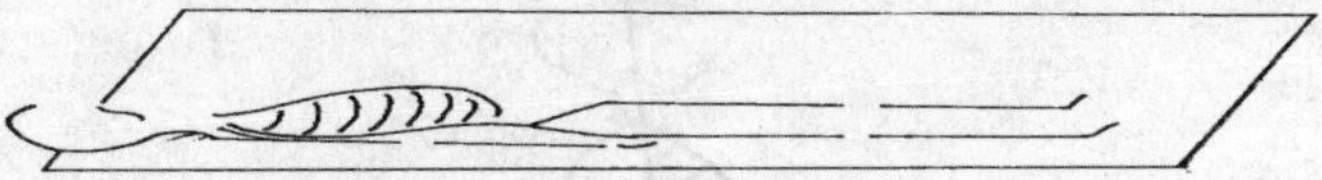

Fig. 4.4: *Fundamental lying position*

Muscle work

- Body is relaxed on a hard surface such as floor or the plinth.
- The head rolls on the side.
- Lumbar spine is hollowed because of the tension of structures lying anterior to the hip joint.
- On soft surfaces such as Mattresses, Spring which way to contour of the body and support it correctly.

- When the lying position is use as a starting position for the exercise it is usually taken on a firm surface.
- The head rotator of both side works reciprocally to stabilize the position of head.
- The extensor of hip and flexor of spine to combat the tendency to hollow the back.
- Medical rotator of hip work to keep the leg in neutral position so that the feet are together.

Effect and uses

- This is an easy position and suitable position for many exercises.
- Breathing is slightly impeded slightly by a pressure on the posterior aspect of thorax.
- Pressure on the abdominal viscera on the surface of diaphragm, often making the position unsuitable for those suffering from respiratory and heart disorder.
- In position hinders return of blood flow from the head and may be unsuitable for elderly person to suffer from high blood pressure.

HANGING POSITION

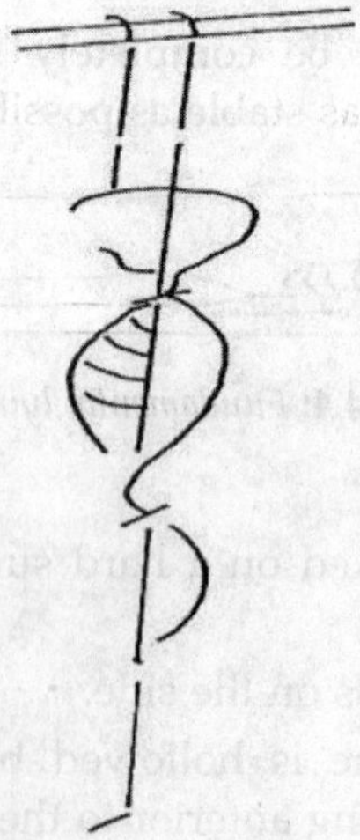

Fig. 4.5: *Fundamental hanging position*

Rules

- Body is supported by grasping on horizontal bar. (Fig. 4.5).
- Forearm being pronated arm straight and shoulder should be wide apart the head is held high and scapula are drawn down and together so that the neck should be elongated.
- The trunk and leg hang straight with the heels together and ankle plantar flexed.

Muscle work

- Flexors of the fingers work strongly to grasp the bar.
- All the muscles round the wrist work strongly to minimize the strain on joint.
- The flexors of elbow works strongly to reduce strain on the joint.
- The adductor of the shoulder works strongly to lift the body on the arms.
- The depressor, retractor of scapula work strongly to fix the scapula and brace the upper back.
- Prevertebral and posterior neck muscle work reciprocally to maintain position of head and neck.
- The abductor of hip work to keep the leg together.
- The extensor of the knee work to keep the leg straight.
- The plantar flexor works to keep the toes face downward.

Effect and uses

- The weight of shoulder taken over the spine and the weight of the leg exert traction upon it.
- It is straighter and elongated.
- The thorax is fixed in the inspiratory position and breathing is difficult and therefore position is difficult for big patient and those suffering from cardiac and respiratory condition.

5

DERIVED POSITION

DEFINITION

Derived positions are altered position of the fundamental position so as to modify the effect of positions or exercises.

PURPOSE

- To increase or decrease the size and stability of the base.
- To raise or lower the centre of gravity.
- To ensure maximum local or general relaxation.
- To alter the position of the body in relation to gravity.
- To provide control or fixation for a particular part of the body so that movement may be localized to specific area.
- To increase or decrease the muscle work required to maintain the position.
- To increase or decrease the leverage.
- To provide a convenient position from which a particular exercise is to be performed.

DERIVED POSITION OF STANDING WITH THE INVOLVEMENT OF LOWER LIMB

Close Standing—Lower portion of legs are close to each other. There is no gap between the feet. (Fig. 5.1).

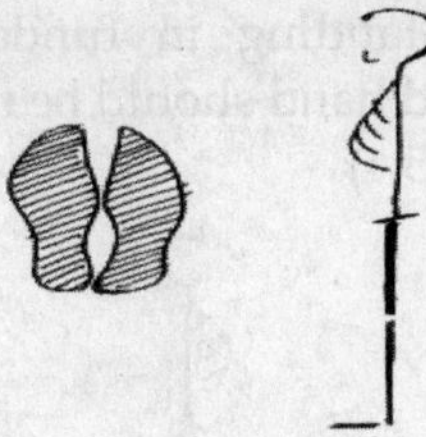

Fig. 5.1: *Close standing*

Toes Standing—Leg should be in fundamental position and stands on toes. (Fig. 5.2).

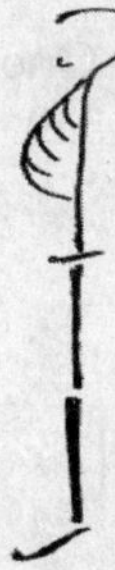

Fig. 5.2: *Toes standing*

Stride Standing—Position should be in fundamental standing and legs are separated from each other. Feet separated from each other to some distance. (Fig. 5.3).

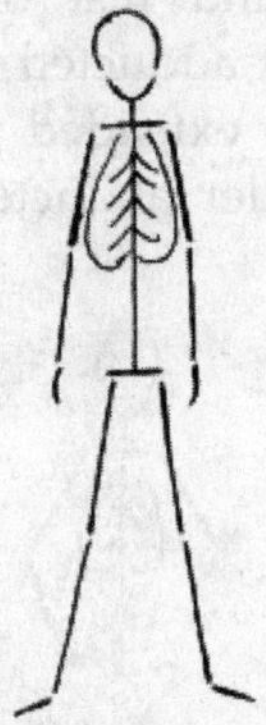

Fig. 5.3: *Stride standing*

Walk Standing—Standing in fundamental position foot your one leg forward and hand should be remains is fundamental standing position. (Fig. 5.4)

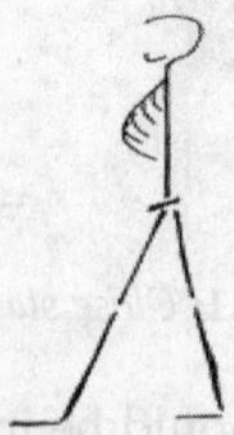

Fig. 5.4: *Walk standing*

Step or Half Standing—One leg should be put on some higher base for stability. (Fig. 5.5).

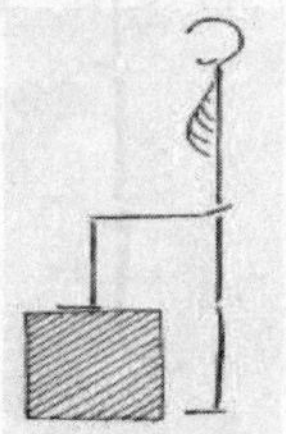

Fig. 5.5: *Step or Half standing*

DERIVED POSITION FROM STANDING WITH INVOLVEMENT OF UPPER LIMB

Wing Standing—Hand rest on the crest of Ilium, the fingers are extended and adducted placed anterior and thumb posteriorly. Wrists are in extended position, forearm pronated, elbow flexed and shoulder abducted and elbow point facing sideways. (Fig. 5.6)

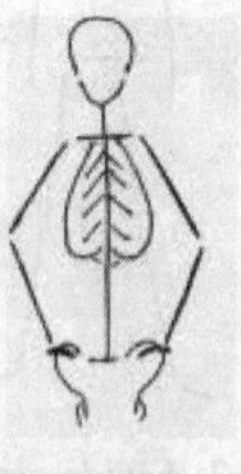

Fig. 5.6: *Wing standing*

Low Wing Standing—Arms are straight and elevated sideways, finger facing downwards, thumbs facing anteriorly and wrist are similar to wing standing. (Fig. 5.7)

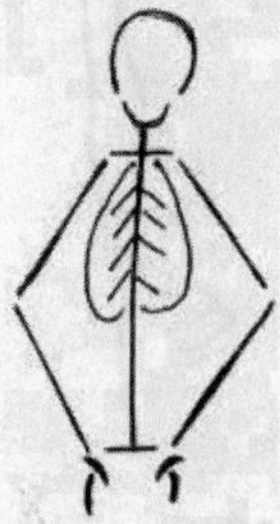

Fig. 5.7: *Low wing standing*

Reach Standing—Both upper arms flex up to 900, palm faces inward and distance between palms is approx half foot. (Fig. 5.8)

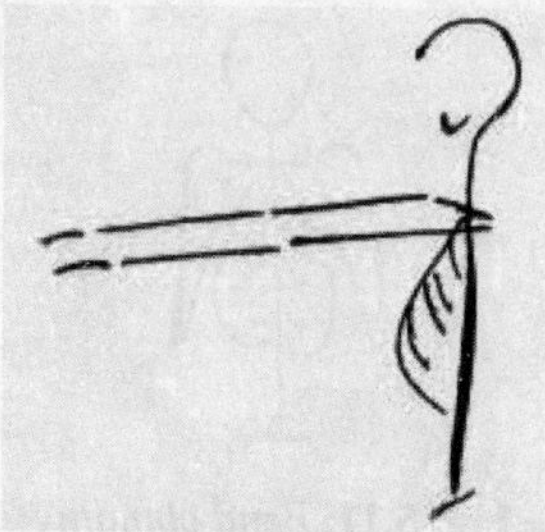

Fig. 5.8: *Reach standing*

Yard Standing—Shoulders are abducted, elbow extended and both arm are parallel to the ground and right angle to the body and palm faces downward. (Fig. 5.9)

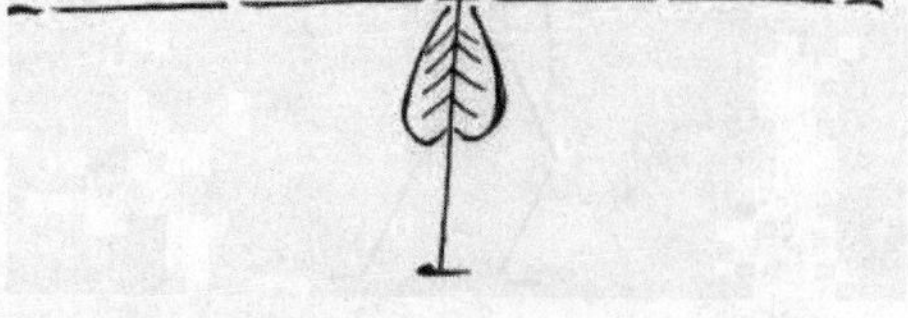

Fig. 5.9: *Yard standing*

Stretch Standing—The arms are fully elevated so that they are in line with the body, parallel to each other and with palm facing inward. (Fig. 5.10)

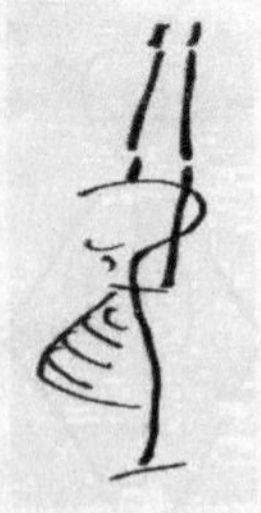

Fig. 5.10: *Stretch standing*

Bend Standing—Shoulder slightly flexed adducted and laterally rotated, elbow fully flexed, wrist and finger slightly flexed. (Fig. 5.11)

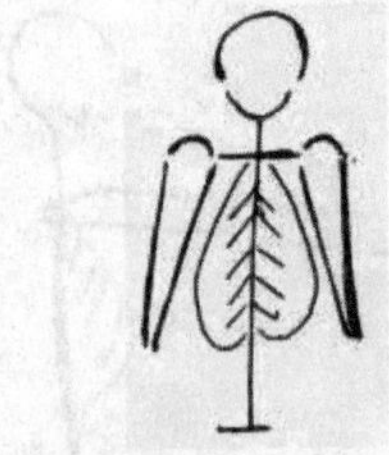

Fig. 5.11: *Bend standing*

Lunge Sideway Standing—Distance between both feet is approx 3 foot. Knee joint of one leg should be bent other leg should be straight and trunk shifted towards the bent knee. (Fig. 5.12)

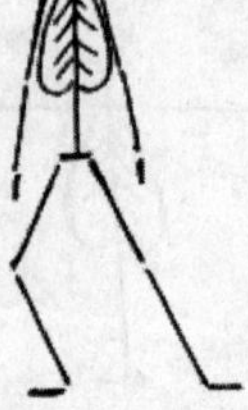

Fig. 5.12: *Lunge sideway standing*

Stoop Standing—A person should be stand is fundamental standing position. Hip joint are flexed while trunk, head and arm remain in alignment and inclined forward. (Fig. 5.13)

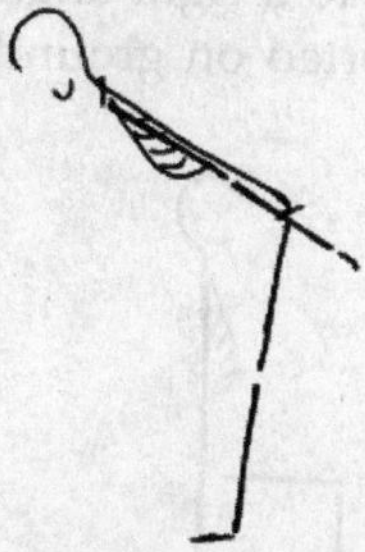

Fig. 5.13: *Stoop standing*

Fallout Standing—One leg is placed directly infront at a distance of three feet and the knees are bend. The back remains straight and body inclined forward. (Fig. 5.14)

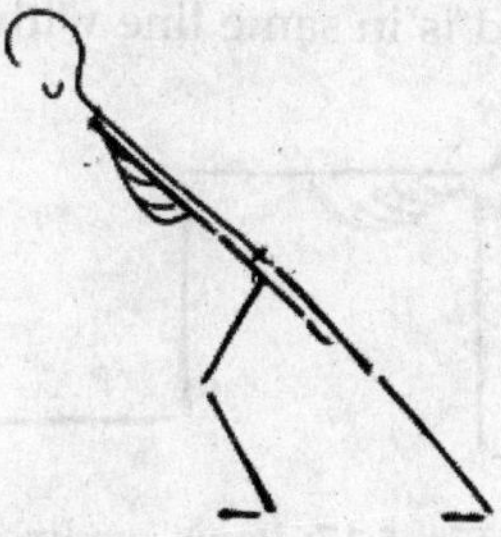

Fig. 5.14: *Fallout standing*

Lax Stoop Standing—The hips are fully flexed and the trunk, head and arm are relaxed so that the hand forward and downward. (Fig. 5.15)

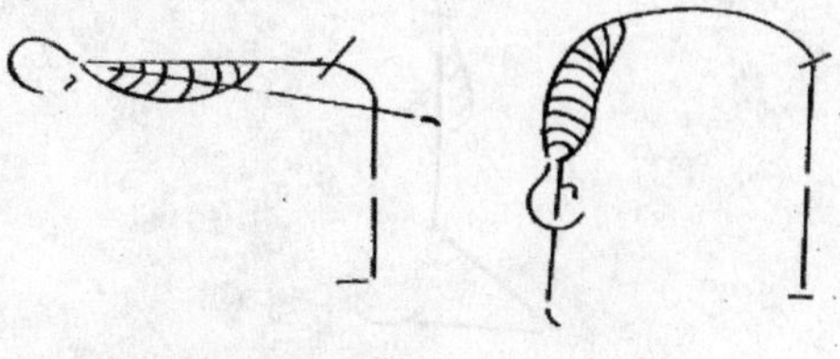

Fig. 5.15: *Lax stoop standing*

DERIVED POSITION OF KNEELING

Half Kneeling—One knee supports most of the body waight and the other leg is bent to a right angle at hip, knee and ankle so that the foot is supported on ground is a forward direction. (Fig. 5.16)

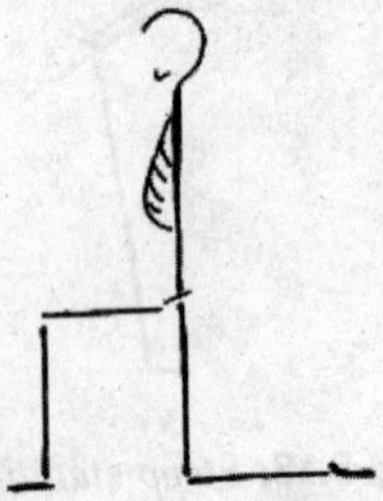

Fig. 5.16: *Half kneeling*

Prone Kneeling—Trunk is horizontal supported under the shoulder by the arms and the pelvis by the thigh which must be held vertical. The head is in same line with the trunk. (Fig. 5.17)

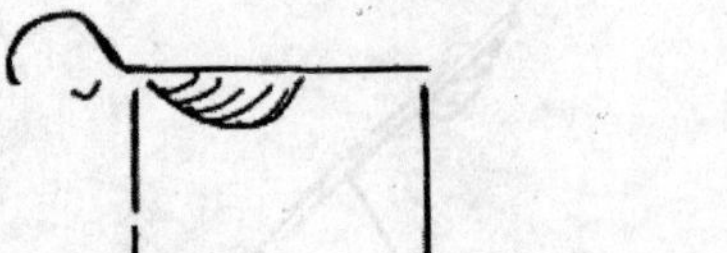

Fig. 5.17: *Prone kneeling*

Kneel Sitting—Knees and hip are flexed so that the person sits on on his knees. The position is some time used for small children the most people find it very uncomfortable. (Fig. 5.18)

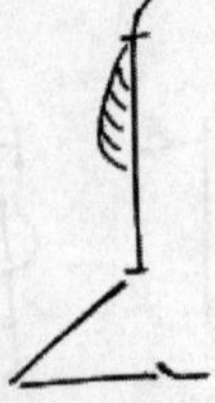

Fig. 5.18: *Kneel sitting*

Inclined Prone Kneeling—This is similar to prone kneeling but the trunk inclined forward and downward and head supported on hand and with elbow flexed. (Fig. 5.19)

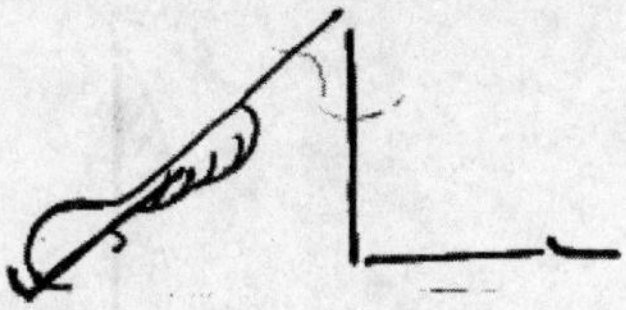

Fig. 5.19: *Inclined prone kneeling*

DERIVED POSITION OF SITTING

Stride Sitting—Similar to fundamental sitting position except that legs are abducted so that feet are two foot apart. (Fig. 5.20)

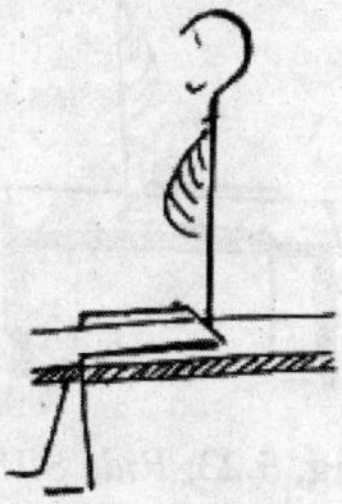

Fig. 5.20: *Stride Sitting*

Crook Sitting—Sitting on plinth with hip and knee flexed and ankle plantar flexed. Feet are together and flat on floor. Knees are either together or apart. (Fig. 5.21)

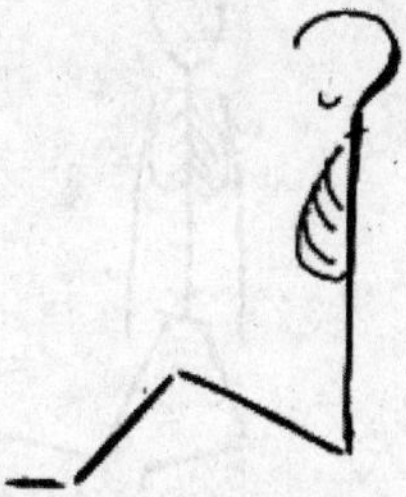

Fig. 5.21: *Crook Sitting*

Long Sitting—Same as crook sitting but knees are extended so that the whole lower limb supported on floor. (Fig. 5.22)

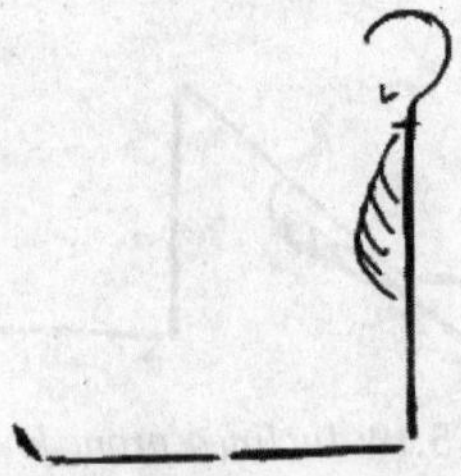

Fig. 5.22: *Long Sitting*

Ride Sitting—Similar to fundamental sitting position, knees fully adducted, flexed is right angle. (Fig. 5.23)

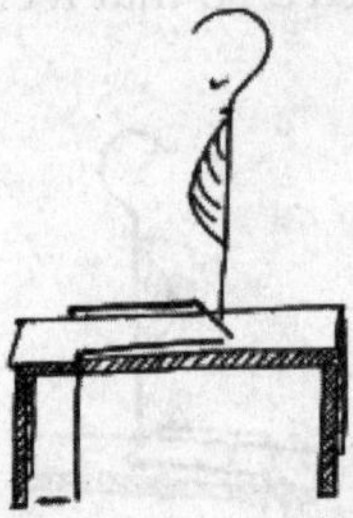

Fig. 5.23: *Ride Sitting*

Side Sitting—Body weight is concentrated on one hip joint, one knee joint is in valgus, flexed and other knee is in varus, flexed. Other hip joint is adducted, flexed and medially rotated. (Fig. 5.24)

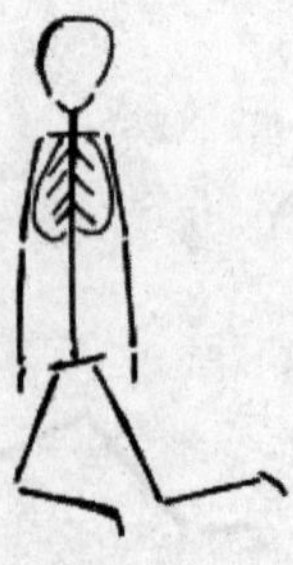

Fig. 5.24: *Side sitting*

Stoop Sitting—It is similar to fundamental sitting position but hip joint flexed forward so trunk region comes forward. (Fig. 5.25)

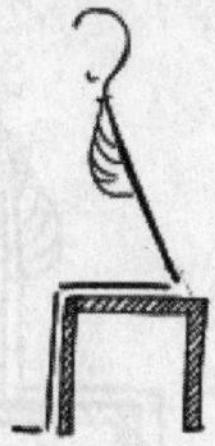

Fig. 5.25: *Stoop sitting*

Fallout Sitting—It is similar to fallout standing sit on a stool and one knee joint is at right angle and other knee and ankle joint is fully extended and the trunk, head and leg are positioned in a line. One hip joint is extended and other joint is flexed. (Fig. 5.26)

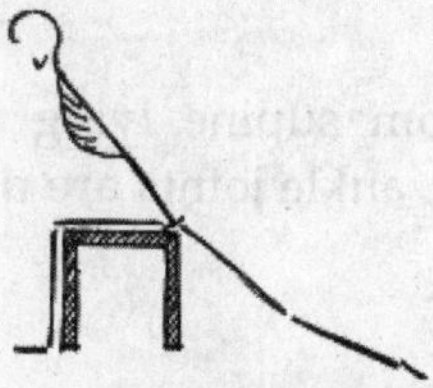

Fig. 5.26: *Fallout sitting*

Cross Sitting—It is similar crook sitting but ankle joints are overlapping each other knees are flexed, hip joints are abducted. Knees are pressed to the floor. (Fig. 5.27)

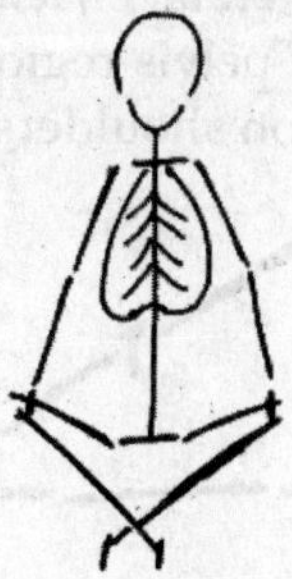

Fig. 5.27: *Cross sitting*

High Sitting—It is similar to fundamental sitting but the legs are off the floor. It is done on high plinth or stool. (Fig. 5.28)

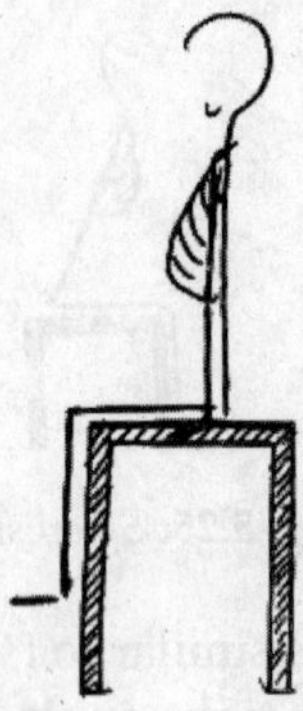

Fig. 5.28: *High Sitting*

DERIVED POSITION FROM LYING WITH INVOLVEMENT OF LEGS

Crook Lying—From supine lying position hip and knee joint are flexed or bent, ankle joints are dorsiflexed. (Fig. 5.29)

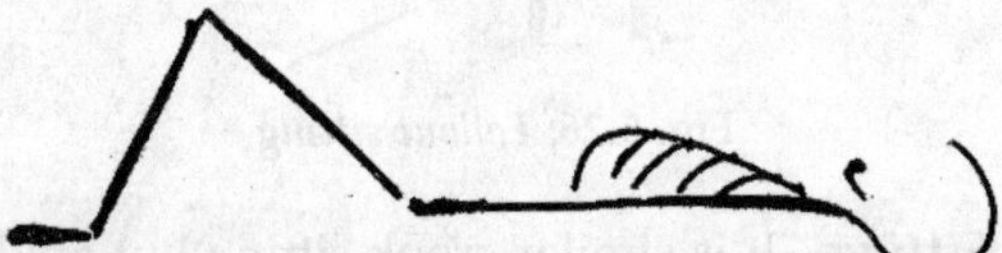

Fig. 5.29: *Crook Lying*

Crook Lying with Pelvis Lifted/Bridging Position—It is similar to crook lying but pelvis region is up or elevated so that the trunk is concentrates on shoulders. (Fig. 5.30)

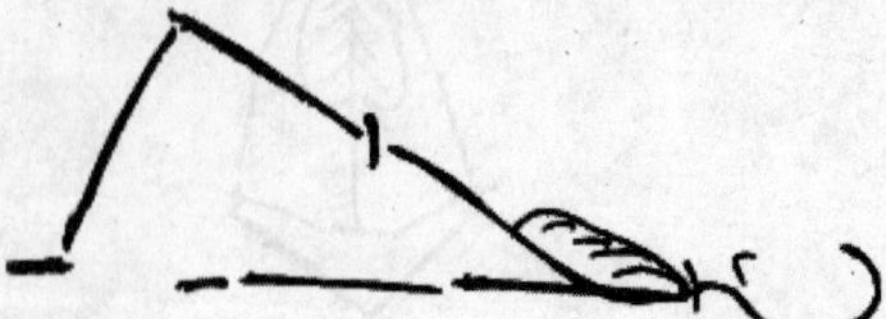

Fig. 5.30: *Crook Lying with Pelvis lifted / bridging position*

Half Lying—In this lying, the legs are straight or horizontal but the trunk region and head is support on oblique base so the hip joint is bent. (Fig. 5.31)

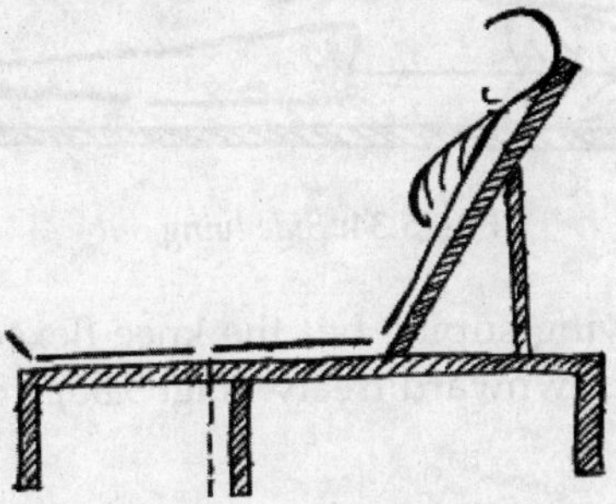

Fig. 5.31: *Half lying*

Prone Lying—In this lying body is erect face facing downwards, body is supported on the floor sole is facing backwards. (Fig. 5.32)

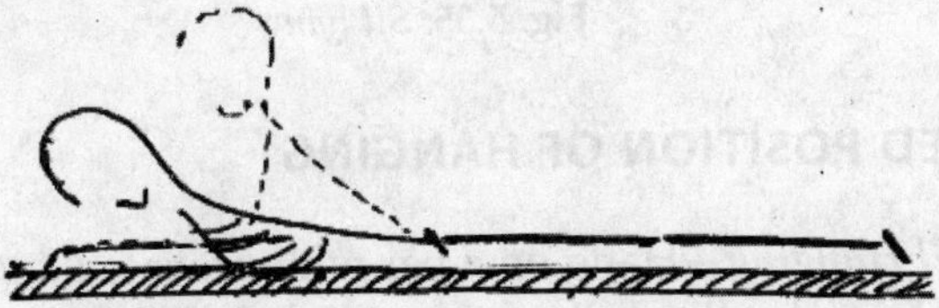

Fig. 5.32: *Prone lying*

Leg Prone Lying—It is similar to prone lying but the trunk and head are not in support of plinth or stool. Anterior parts of legs are supported only. (Fig. 5.33)

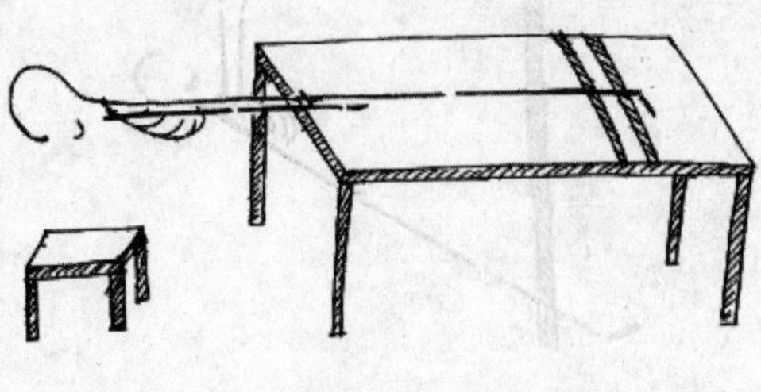

Fig. 5.33: *Leg prone lying*

Side Lying—Lying on the support of side of body. Body is erect and upper leg is placed over lower leg. (Fig. 5.34)

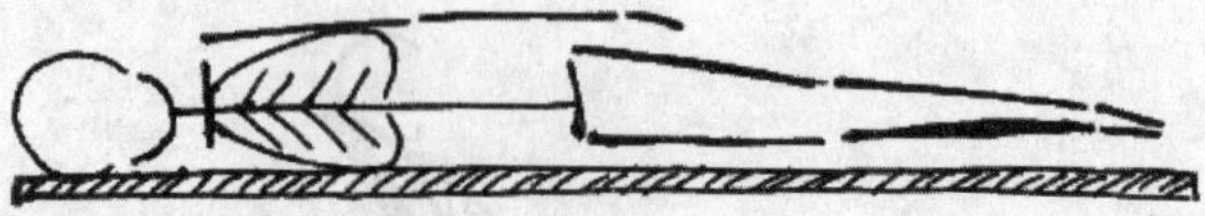

Fig. 5.34: *Side lying*

Sit Lying—Lying supine but the knee flexed at right angle and legs hanging downward freely. (Fig. 5.35)

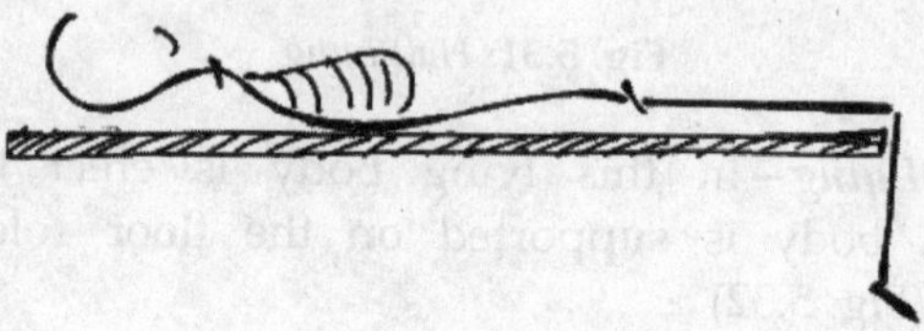

Fig. 5.35: *Sit lying*

DERIVED POSITION OF HANGING

Fall Hanging—Hang on a bar with pronated and hands are parallel to each other, elbow is extended. Arm joint are flexed, head, trunk and legs are is line. Body and arms are at right angle. (Fig. 5.36)

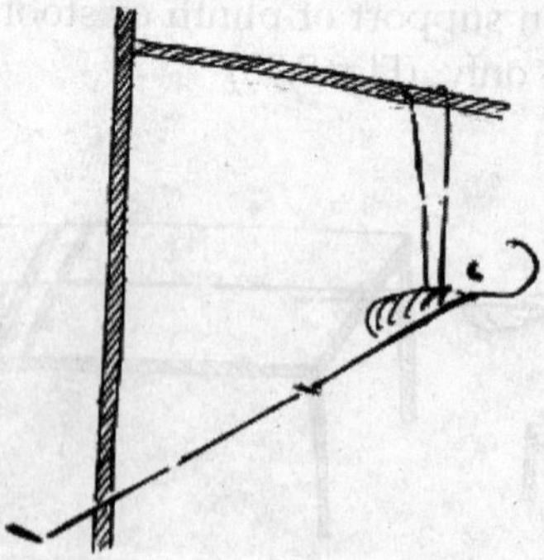

Fig. 5.36: *Fall hanging* (Fig. 5.36)

SPECIALLY DERIVED POSITION

Crouch Sitting—Hip and knee joint are fully flexed, trunk is straight and hand is in resting position to floor, mostly weight of body concentrated on toes. Ankle joint is flexed. (Fig. 5.37)

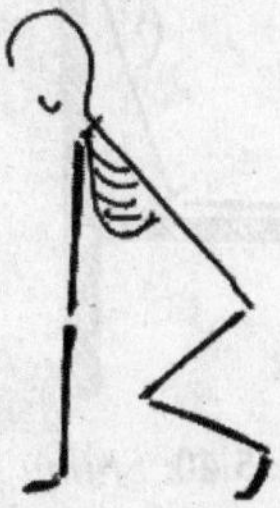

Fig. 5.37: *Crouch sitting*

Prone Falling—Head, trunk and legs are in line. Hands are situated vertically to the body for support and ankle joint are fully flexed. Some body weight is concentrated on toes. (Fig. 5.38)

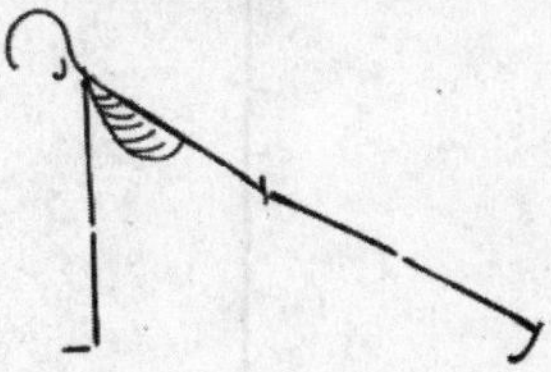

Fig. 5.38: *Prone falling*

Side Falling—Head, trunk, legs and one hand are a line. One hand is vertically arranged to the body for support. One hip joint is slightly bent. (Fig. 5.39)

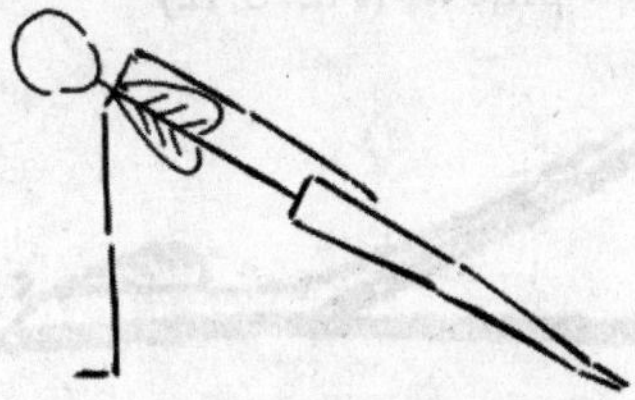

Fig. 5.39: *Side falling*

Slump Sitting—Sit on a chair without full support of back bone or spine. Spine is bent. (Fig. 5.40)

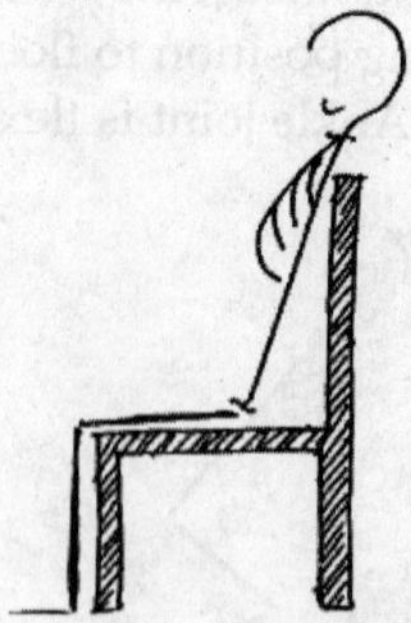

Fig. 5.40: *Slump sitting*

Heel Standing—Erect stand on the heel. (Fig. 5.41)

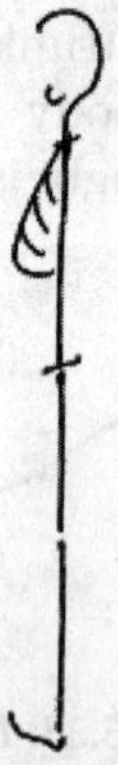

Fig. 5.41: *Heel standing*

Leg Elevated Lying—Lying supine with bent the hip joint so that the leg is elevated. Knee joint fully extended. Mostly elevated legs put on pillow. (Fig. 5.42)

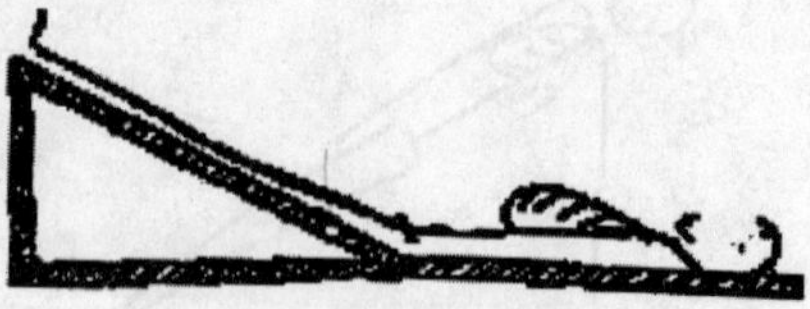

Fig. 5.42: *Leg elevated lying*

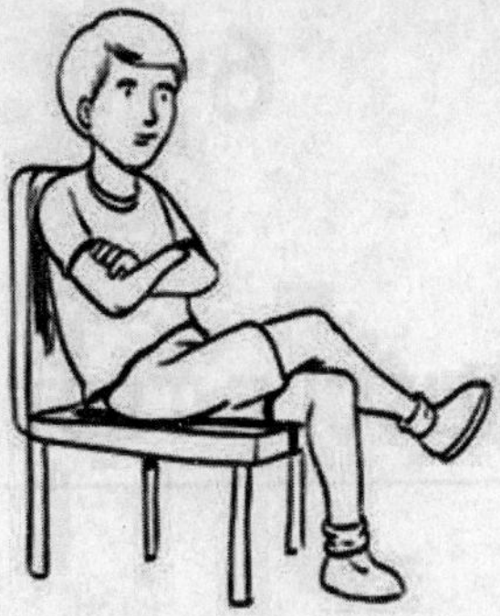

Fig. 5.43: *Cross chair sitting*

Cross Chair Sitting **–** Sit on a chair. One leg is in fundamental position but one leg's knee overlap or cross to another leg's knee. (Fig. 5.43)

6

MANUAL MUSCLE TESTING (MMT)

INTRODUCTION

1. Muscle testing is the integral part of physical examination. It provides information that is useful in differential diagnosis, Prognosis, treatment of neuromuscular and musculoskeletal disorders.
2. The care must be given for injured part and the patient should be in comfortable position to avoid discomfort and pain. Gentle touch is requiring during muscles testing for very weak muscle.
3. Is muscle testing done for strength?
4. All these type of testing are the parts of muscle testing based on experience.
5. Cause of treatment of weak muscle – Muscle weakness should be treated by treating the basic cause of weakness such as –
   - If weakness due to lack of use – Then give exercise
   - If weakness due to overworks and fatigue – Then give rest
   - If weakness due to stretch and strain – Then relief of stress and strain by avoiding the exercise and stress or additional exercise is thrust (affect) upon the weak muscle
   - Two muscles in the body are having net exactly function but if any one muscle got injured/paralyzed then mobility and stability of the part will also be impaired. The treat the paralyzed/ injured muscle accordingly.

- If excessive shortening of muscle , contracture occurs, this can also leads to impairment, then treat the contracture and shortening.

FUNDAMENTAL COMPONENTS OF MMT

There are two fundamental component of MMT:

1. The test performance
2. Evaluation

The Test Performance

To know about the grade of paralysis and grade of muscle strength, prolonged experience and detail knowledge about muscle function the practice is necessary to acquired it by skill in performing the grading of muscle strength.

Evaluation

In condition of muscle testing primarily, the musculoskeletal evaluation should be done then evaluation fairly diagnosed.

PRINCIPALS OF MMT

Determined the muscle to check treated the muscle weakness some ways followed as –

1. Determined the muscle which will be under testing, then test it carefully and make a chart about the grasp of muscle which will be treated and also the part of each muscle, degree of each muscle
2. Insist the patient for discipline and also make a privacy between patient and physiotherapist by these, patient can give the cooperation and undivided attention
3. Use some preliminary (starting, warming up exercise in some case like cyanosis, muscle, weakness etc)
4. Supporting the treating part
5. Free from covering / expose the treating part

CRITERIA OF MUSCLES TESTING

- Oxford classification based on performance of muscle action. Before going to assess examiner have full idea of anatomy, physiology, pathology, biomechanics and other associated condition.
- MMT is used in finding out the degree of weakening or a particular muscle in various conditions like injury, paralysis and other musculoskeletal dysfunction.
- In some conditions, MMT cannot be performed. E.g. - Mad person, mentally retarded person, spastic child, neonatal child, person is in coma, person with high fever.

Indications

- Hemiplegia
- Paraplegia
- Monoplegia
- Quadriplegia
- Diplegia
- Brachial plexus injury
- Weakness due to cervical spondylosis
- Iatrogenic
- Saturday night paralysis
- Carpel tunnel syndrome
- Bell's Palsy
- Post Traumatic weakness
- G.B. Syndrome
- Muscular dystrophy
- Laterally palpated valve injury
- Weakness in L/E due to PIVD (prolapse intervertebral disc)
- Hensen's disease.

Contraindications

- Open injury
- Severe spasticity
- Fracture

- Subluxation and dislocation
- Hemophilia
- Osteomyelitis
- Immediately after surgery
- Cardiovascular conditions
- Abnormal hernia

Grading of Muscles

Rule of numerical grading system for muscle strength

0. No palpable or no visual contraction.
1. Trace muscle contraction is palpable; no body part motion is considered.
2. Full range of motion with gravity eliminated plane.
3. Full range of motion is present against gravity without resistance.
4. Full range of motion is present against gravity with considerable resistance to motion provided by examiner.
5. Full range of motion is present against gravity with strong resistance to motion provided by examiner.

(+) and (-) symbols can be used to provide finer discrimination between the above criteria, as:-

- **Zero (0/5):** The subject demonstrates no palpable muscle contraction.
- **Trace (1/5):** The subject's muscle contraction can be palpated, but there is no joint movement.
- **Poor Minus (2-/5):** The subject does not complete range of motion with gravity eliminated position.
- **Poor (2/5):** The subject does not complete range of motion with gravity eliminated.
- **Poor Plus (2+/5):** The subject does not complete range of motion against gravity.
- **Fair Minus (3-/5):** The subject does not complete range of motion against gravity, but does complete more than half of the range.

- **Fair (3/5):** The subject completes range of motion against gravity without manual resistance.
- **Fair Plus (3+/5):** The subject completes range of motion against gravity with only minimal resistance.
- **Good Minus (4-/5):** The subject completes range of motion against gravity with minimal-moderate resistance.
- **Good (4/5):** The subject completes range of motion against gravity with moderate resistance.
- **Good Plus (4+/5):** The subject completes range of motion against gravity with moderate-maximal resistance.
- **Normal (5/5):** The subject completes range of motion against gravity with maximum resistance.

MMT of Knee Extensors

Muscles of knee extensors: Quadriceps (Rectus femoris, vastus lateralis, vastus medialis, vastus intermedius).

Grade 0: Muscle is fully paralyzed. No muscle contraction after visual inspection or palpation. Patient is in supine lying position and contraction of quadriceps determined by palpation or visual inspection of tendon between patella and tuberosity of tibia and muscle fibers. (Fig. 6.1)

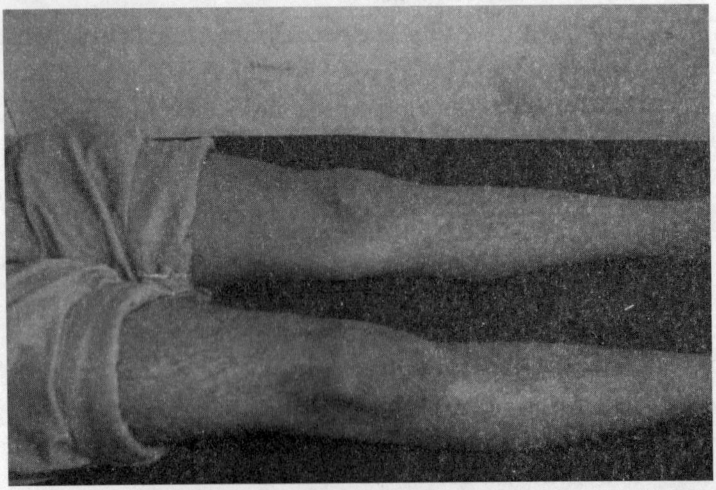

Fig. 6.1: *Grade 0 (No visual contraction)*

Grade 1 – Patient is inside lying position with testing limb downward. Testing knee should be in flexed position. No movement but flicker of contraction can be palpated by placing the hand over muscle belly as the patient tries to perform the movement. (Fig. 6.2).

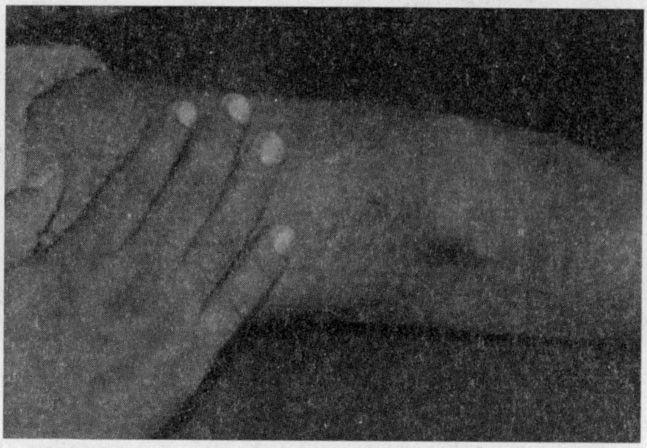

Fig. 6.2: *Grade 1 – Flicker of contraction*

Grade 2 – Patient is in side lying position with testing limb downward. Testing knee should be in flexed position. In gravity eliminated position full range of motion available at knee joint. (Fig. 6.3).

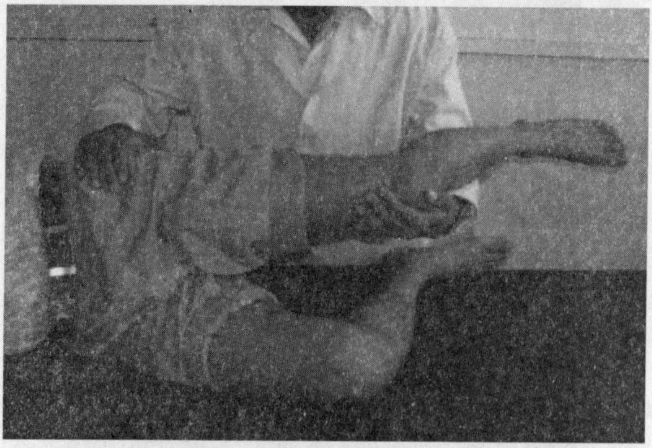

Fig. 6.3: *Grade 2- Full range of motion in gravity eliminated position*

Grade 3 – Patient is in high sitting position. Full range of motion available at knee joint against gravity without any external resistance. Therapist will stabilize the proximal part of the joint by the hand. (Fig. 6.4).

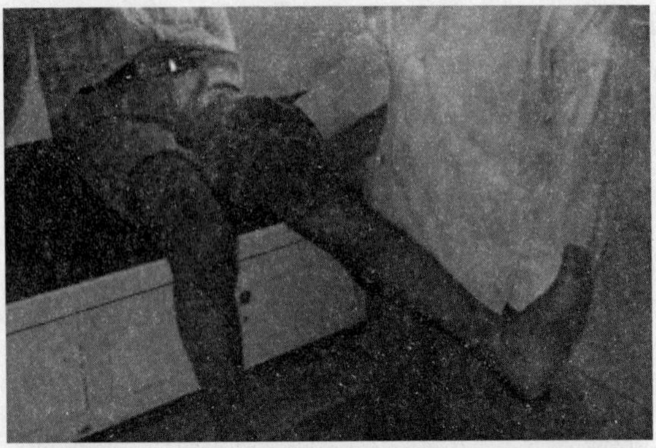

Fig. 6.4: *Grade 3- full range of motion against gravity*

Grade 4 and 5 - Patient is in high sitting position. Full range of motion available at knee joint against gravity with external resistance. In grade 4 moderate resistances will be required but in grade 5 maximum resistances will be required. Stabilize thigh above the knee joint (by the therapist). Resistance is given just above the ankle joint. (Fig. 6.5).

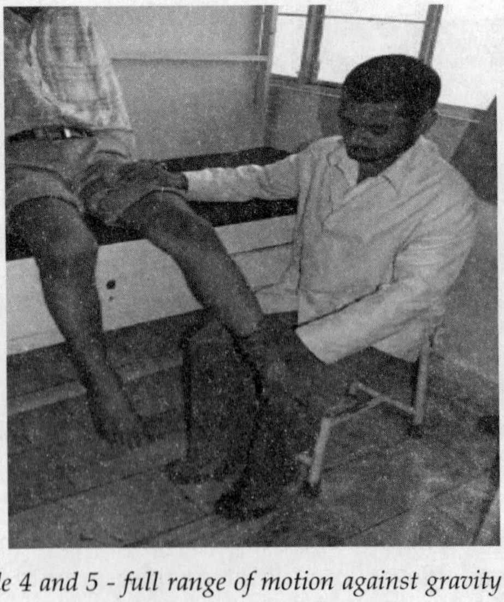

Fig. 6.5: *Grade 4 and 5 - full range of motion against gravity with moderate and maximum resistance*

MMT PERFORMA

Patient Name :.................................... Address :...........................

Age/Sex :..Onset :..........................

ID Number :..

Date of Examination :...

Examiner's Name :..

LEFT			Date of Examination / Examiner's Name		RIGHT		
3	2	1			1	2	3
			NECK				
				Capital extension			
				Cervical extension			
				Combined extension (capital plus cervical)			
				Capital flexion			
				Cervical flexion			
				Combined flexion (capital plus cervical)			
				Combined flexion and rotation (Sternocleidomastoid)			
				Cervical rotation			
			TRUNK				
				Extension – Lumbar			
				Extension – Thoracic			
				Pelvic elevation			
				Flexion			
				Rotation			
				Diaphragm strength			
				Maximal inspiration less or full expiration (indirect intercostals test) (inches)			
				Cough (indirect forced expiration)			

LEFT			Date of Examination / Examiner's Name		RIGHT		
3	2	1			1	2	3
			UPPER EXTREMITY				
			Shoulder Joint	Scapular abduction and upward rotation			
				Scapular elevation			
				Scapular adduction			
				Scapular adduction and down-ward rotation			
				Shoulder flexion			
				Shoulder extension			
				Shoulder adduction			
				Shoulder abduction			
				Shoulder horizontal abduction			
				Shoulder horizontal adduction			
				Shoulder external rotation			
				Shoulder internal rotation			
			Elbow Joint	Elbow flexion			
				Elbow extension			
			Forearm Motions	Forearm Supination			
				Forearm Pronation			
			Wrist Joint	Wrist flexion			
				Wrist extension			
			MCP Joint	Finger metacarpophalangeal flexion			
				Finger proximal interphalangeal flexion			
				Finger distal interphalangeal flexion			
				Finger metacarpophalangeal extension			

LEFT			Date of Examination / Examiner's Name		RIGHT		
3	2	1			1	2	3
				Finger abduction			
				Finger adduction			
			Thumb	Thumb metacarpophalangeal flexion			
				Thumb interphalangeal flexion			
				Thumb metacarpophalangeal extension (motion superior to plane of metacarpals)			
				Thumb interphalangeal extension			
				Thumb carpometacarpal abduction (motion perpendicular to plane of palm)			
				Thumb carpometacarpal abduction and extension (motion parallel to plane of palm)			
				Thumb CMC joint adduction			
				Thumb opposition			
				Little finger opposition			
			LOWER EXTREMITY				
			Hip Joint	Hip flexion			
				Hip extension (Gluteus maximus)			
				Hip abduction			
				Hip abduction			
				Hip external rotation			
				Hip internal rotation			
			Knee Joint	Knee flexion			
				Knee flexion with leg external rotation			

LEFT			Date of Examination / Examiner's Name		RIGHT		
3	2	1			1	2	3
				Knee flexion with leg internal rotation			
				Knee extension			
			Ankle Joint	Ankle plantar flexion			
				Ankle plantar flexion (soleus)			
				Foot dorsiflexion and inversion			
				Foot inversion			
				Foot eversion with plantar flexion			
				Foot eversion with dorsiflexion			
			Toes	Great toe metatarsophalangeal flexion			
				Toe metatarsophalangeal flexion			
				Great toe interphalangeal flexion			
				Toe interphalangeal flexion			
				Great toe metatarsohalangeal extension			
				Toe metatarsophalangeal extension			
				Great toe interphalangeal extension			
				Toe interphalangeal extension			

Comments:

....

....

....

....

....

....

Diagnosis ....

onset ....

Examiner/Physiotherepist Name ....

7

GONIOMETRY

INTRODUCTION

The term goniometry is derived from two Greek words; Gonia means Angle and Metron means Measure. Therefore goniometry refers to the measurement of angles created at human joints by the bones of the body. Goniometry is an assessment tools which measure the total amount of motion available at joint. (Fig. 7.1 and Fig. 7.2).

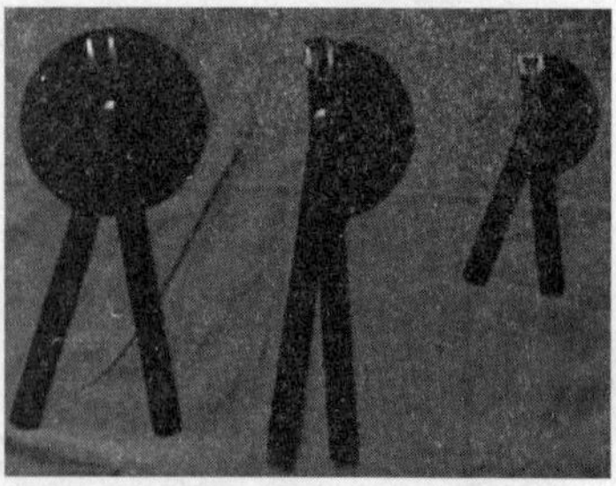

Fig. 7.1: *Different goniometers*

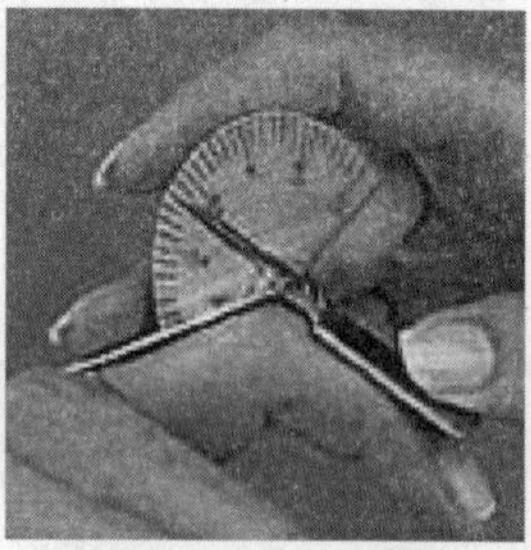

Fig. 7.2: *Finger Goniometer*

RANGE OF MOTION

The amount of motion that is available a joint is called range of motion (ROM). There are lots of factors affecting range of motion like age, gender, pain etc. Active range of motion (AROM) refers to the amount of joint motion attained by a subject during unassisted voluntary joint motion. Passive joint of motion (PROM) is the amount of motion attained by an examiner without assistance from the subject.

Range of Motion for Upper Limb

1. ***Shoulder Joint***
   Flexion – 0 – 180° (Flexion – 90° & Hyper flexion – 180°)
   Extension – 180° – 0°
   Hyperextension – 0 – 60°
   Abduction – 0 – 180 ° (Abduction – 90° & Hyper abduction – 170°
   Adduction – 180° – 0 °
   Medial Rotation – 0 – 60 ° or 70°
   Lateral Rotation – 0 – 80 ° or 90°
   Horizontal Abduction – 130°
2. ***Elbow Joint***
   Flexion – 0 – 150°
   Extension – 150° – 0°
3. **Superior Radioulnar Joint**
   Supination – 0 – 80° or 90°
   Pronation – 0 – 80° or 90°
4. ***Wrist Joint***
   Flexion – 0 – 80°
   Extension – 0 – 70°
   Radial deviation – 0 – 20°
   Ulnar Deviation – 0 – 30°
5. ***MCP Joint***
   Flexion – 0 – 80° or 90°
   Extension – 15 – 45° (Hyperextension)
6. ***CMC Joint***
   Adduction – 0 – 50°
   Abduction – 50 – 0°
   Flexion – 0 – 50°
   Extension – 50 – 0°

Range of Motion for Lower Limb

1. ***Hip Joint***
   Flexion – 0 – 80° or 90° (with knee extended)
   Extension – 0 – 135° or 145° – 0°
   Abduction – 0 – 30° or 40°
   Adduction – 0 – 15°
   Lateral Rotation – 0 – 30°
   Medical Rotation – 0 – 45°

2. ***Knee Joint***

Flexion	– 0 – 135° or 145°
Extension	– 135° or 145° – 0°
Medial rotation	– 0 – 80°
Lateral rotation	– 0 – 90°

3. ***Ankle Joint***

Dorsiflexion	– 0 – 20°
Planter flexion	– 0 – 30 or 40°
Inversion	– 0 – 15° or 20°
Eversion	– 10 – 18°

Range of Motion for Cervical Joint

Flexion	– 0– 45°
Extension	– 0 – 30 or 40°
Lateral Rotation	– 0 – 15° or 20°

PROCEDURE FOR GONIOMETRIC MEASUREMENT

The examiner must have knowledge regarding the testing position, alternate position, stabilization required joint, structure and function, anatomical bony landmarks and instruments alignment. As for example ROM measurement for hip lateral rotation Position is high sitting, Axis should be placed at the centre of Patella, Static arm perpendicular to the ground and movable arm parallel to the shine of Tibia. (Fig. 7.3A and 7.3B).

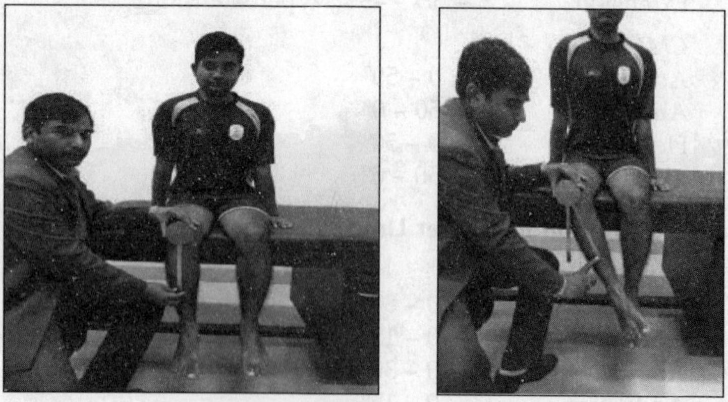

A B

Fig. 7.3: *Method of ROM measurement by Goniometer for hip rotation*

Upper Limb

1. *Shoulder Joint*
   - Flexion and Extension

     Axis – ½ inch below to acromion process (laterally).

     Static bar- Parallel to the trunk.

     Movable bar - Parallel to the lateral epicondyle
   - Adduction and Abduction

     Axis – Posterior part of acromion process

     Static Arm – Parallel to the trunk

     Movable Arm – Parallel to the humerous & olecranon process
   - Horizontal Adduction and Abduction

     Axis – Posterior part of olecranon process

     Static Arm – Parallel to the trunk

     Movable Arm – Parallel to the humerus and Olecranon process
   - Medial and lateral rotation

     Axis – On Olecranon process

     Static Arm – Perpendicular to body

     Movable Arm – Parallel to ulnar border

2. *Elbow Joint*
   - Flexion and Extension

     Axis – Lat epicondyle of Humerus

     Static Arm – Parallel to humerus

     Movable Arm – Parallel to the radius

3. *Superior Radio Ulnar Joint*
   - Supination and Pronation (In Supination – Palmer aspect)

     Axis – Styloid process of ulna on dorsal aspect

     Static Arm – Perpendicular to the ground

     Movable Arm – Parallel to Wrist

4. *Wrist Joint*
   - Extension

     Axis – Base of 2nd M.C. Bone

Static Arm – Parallel to radius

Movable Arm – Parallel to 2nd M.C. bone

This is performed when thumb is position of opposition

- Adduction and Abduction

  Axis – On the base of 3rd M.C. Bone

  Static Arm – Parallel to between radius and Ulna

  Movable Arm – 3rd M.C. Bone one hand should be pronated

5. *Carpometacarpal Joint*

- Adduction and Abduction

  Axis – Between the base of 1st and 2nd M.C. Bone

  Movable Arm – Parallel to first M.C. Bone

  Static Arm – Parallel to radius

- Flexion and Extension

  Axis – Dorsal aspect of M.C. joint

  Static bar – Dorsal aspect of M.C. joint (parallel)

  Movable Arm – On the phalanges

- Abduction of finger

  Axis – M.C.P. joint

  Static Arm – Towards the carpel

  Movable Arm – Over the phalanx

  Hand in prone Position

Lower Limb

1. *Hip Joint*

- Extension

  Position – Prone Lying and knee extension

  Axis – Greater trochanter

  Static Arm – Parallel to the trunk

  Movable Arm – Parallel to the femur

- Flexion

  Position – Supine lying with hip and knee flexion

  Axis – On the greater trochanter

  Static Arm – Parallel to the trunk

Movable Arm – Parallel to the femur (lat side)

- Abduction and Adduction

  Position – Supine lying

  Axis – A.S.I.S. (Ipsilateral)

  Static Arm – Towards opposite A.S.I.S

  Movable Arm - Parallel to femur (ant side of thigh)

- Hip Rotation (lat and med)

  Position – sitting

  Axis – Centre of Patella

  Static Arm – perpendicular to the ground

  Movable Arm – Parallel to the shin of Tibia

2. Knee Joint

Position – prone Lying

Axis – lateral condyle of femur

Static Arm – Parallel to femur

Movable Arm – Parallel to Fibula

3. Ankle Joint

- Dorsiflexion and planter flexion

  Position – Supine lying and sitting

  Axis – 1 ½ inch below the medial maleollus

  Static Arm – Parallel to Tibia

  Movable Arm – Parallel to first metatarsal bone

4. Subtalar Joint

- Eversion and Inversion

  Position – Supine lying or sitting

  Axis – lateral border of Metatarsal bone

  Static Arm – Parallel to tibia

  Movable Arm – Parallel to sole

Cervical Spine

- Flexion and extension

  Position – sitting

  Axis – External auditory meatus

Static Arm – perpendicular to the ground

Movable Arm – base of the nostril

Tape measurement–Distance between tips of the chin to sternal notch (mouth remains close). On tape measurement differences are as-

a. Flexion difference - About 3 inch
b. Extension difference – about 3 inch

- Lateral Flexion

  Position – Back supported sitting

  Axis – C7 vertebrae

  Static Arm – Aligned with thoracic vertebrae

  Movable Arm – Dorsal mid line of the head

  Tape measurement– Mastoid Process to Coracoid process

- Rotation

  Position - sitting (thoracic and lumber vertebrae

  Axis – Over the centre of cranial aspect of head

  Static Arm - Align with the tip of the nose

  Tape measurement- Tip of chin to acromion process

■

8

THERAPEUTIC GYMNASIUM

EXERCISE THERAPY LAB EQUIPMENT WITH DIAGRAMMATIC REPRESENTATION

1. Ankle Exerciser

- Improve ROM at the ankle joint.
- For strengthening of planter flexor muscles of ankle. (Fig. 8.1).

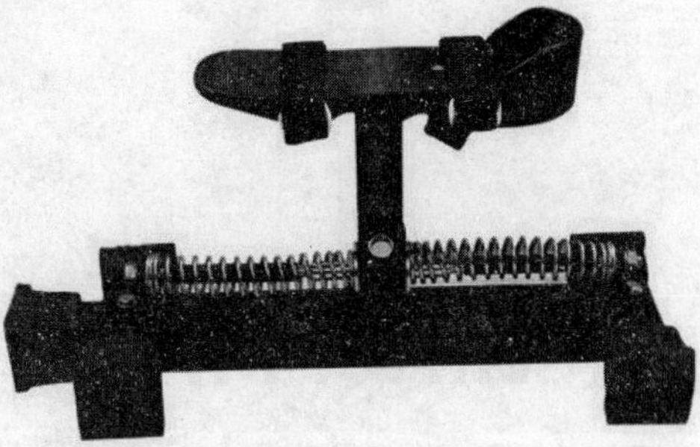

Fig. 8.1: *Ankle exerciser*

2. Heel Exerciser

- To improve the ROM at ankle joint and other associate joint of foot.
- Improve dorsiflexion or planterflexion at ankle joint
- Improve stabilization at ankle. (Fig. 8.2).

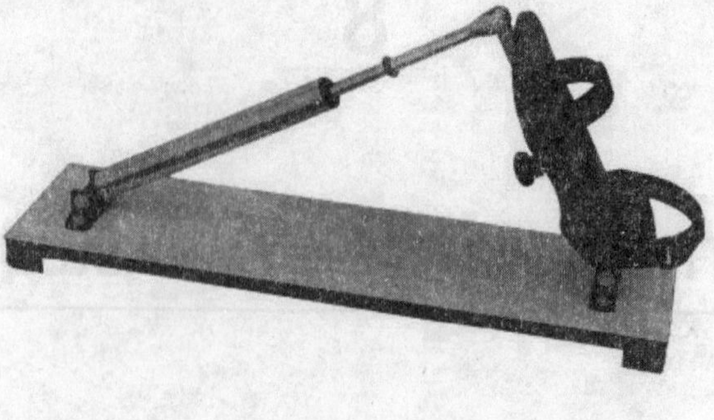

Fig. 8.2: *Heal exerciser*

3. Axillary Crutch

- To provide the support during walking.
- Used in gait training. (Fig. 8.3).

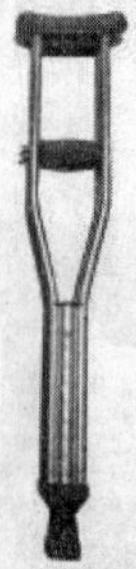

Fig. 8.3: *Axillary crutch*

4. Elbow Exerciser

- Improve ROM at elbow joint.
- For strengthening of muscle around the elbow joint.
- Improve the stabilization of Elbow joint.

5. Finger Ladder

- Improve ROM of flexion and abduction of shoulder joint.
- Strengthening of whole upper limb. (Fig. 8.4).

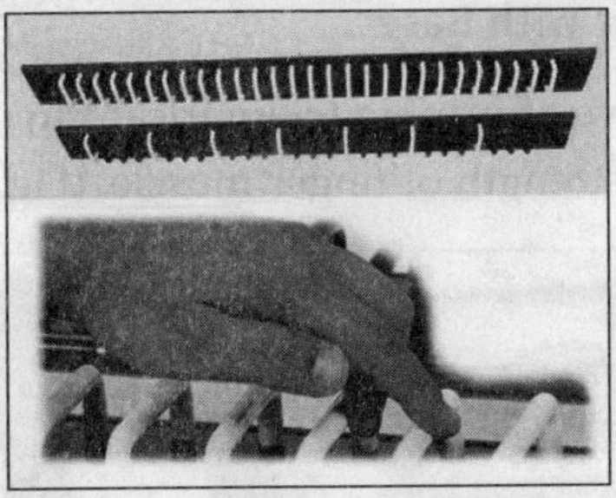

Fig. 8.4: *Finger ladder*

6. Thera Band

- This is ideal for upper and lower body conditioning.
- It improves strength, Coordination of muscle. (Fig. 8.5).

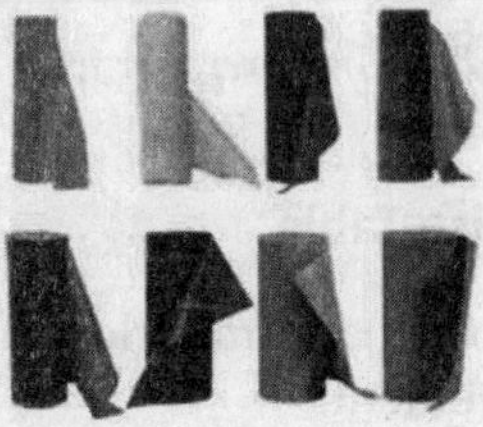

Fig. 8.5: *Thera band*

7. Goniometer

- To measure the ROM
- To assess the improvement of the treatment given at the joint. (Fig. 8.6).

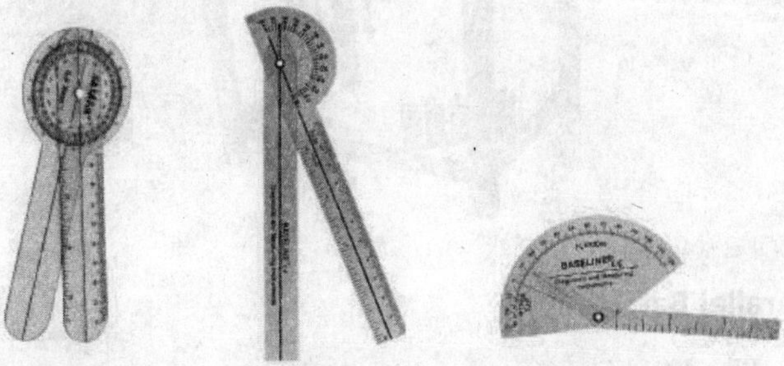

Full Circle   Half Circle   Finger

Fig. 8.6: *Goniometer*

8. Grip Exerciser with Base

- To improve of griping (cylindrical, circular)
- Improve strength of finger muscle. (Fig. 8.7).

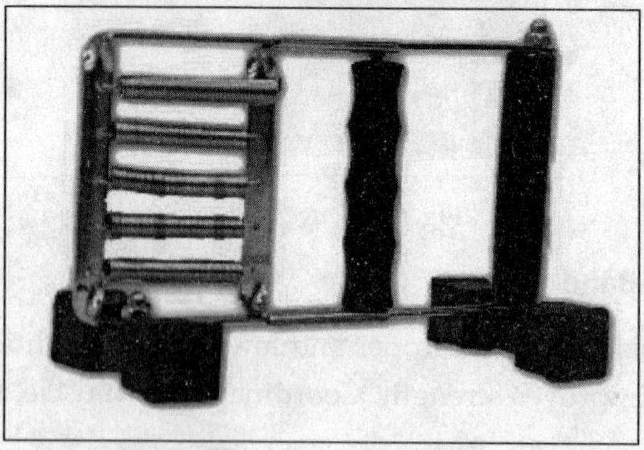

Fig. 8.7: *Grip exerciser with base*

9. Multi Hand Exercise Table

- To strengthen the hand muscles and muscles responsible for finger movement.
- Improve ROM of fingers and wrist.
- Improve fine movement of finger.

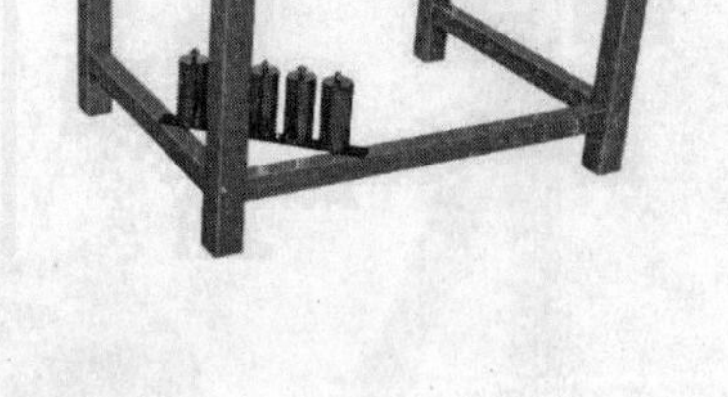

10. Parallel Bar

- Used to give proper gait training
- Progressive weight bearing.

- To provide gait training with orthotic and prosthetic devices (Amputation). (Fig. 8.8).

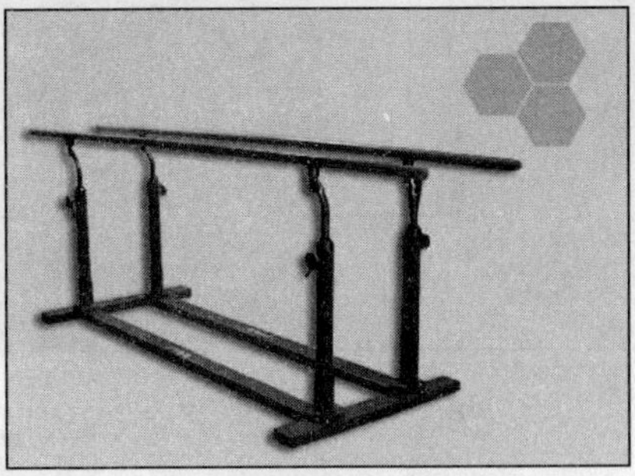

Fig. 8.8: *Parallel Bar*

11. Ramp and Stair Exerciser

- Strengthen Quadriceps and hamstring
- Improve walking
- Improve balance. (Fig. 8.9).

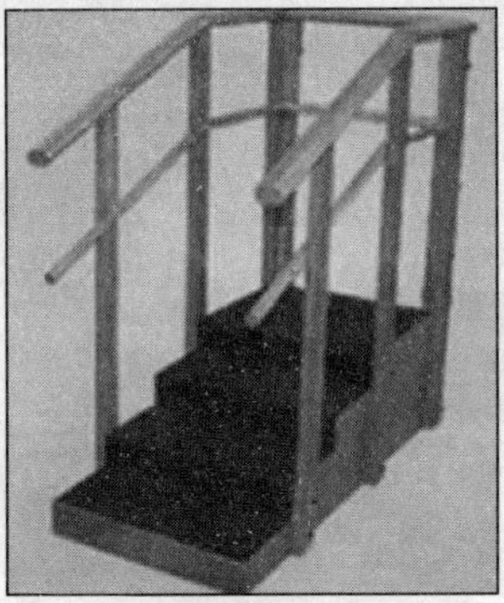

Fig. 8.9: *Ramp and stair exerciser*

12. Shoulder Wheel

- To Improve ROM of Shoulder joints
- Break the adhesion of shoulder joints
- Provide relaxation of muscle around the shoulder joint. (Fig. 8.10).

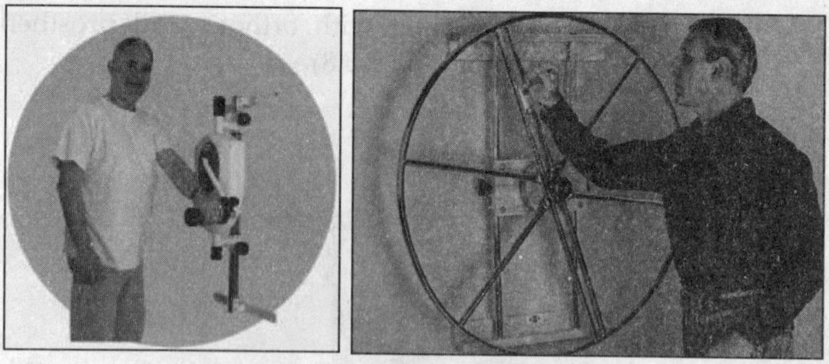

Fig. 8.10: *Shoulder wheel*

13. Stepper

- Training machine on which movement Similar to running are performed.
- It strengthens the quadriceps, hamstring and calf muscle.
- It is usually set at a lower level for developing aerobic fitness but should be higher to develop endurance. (Fig. 8.11).

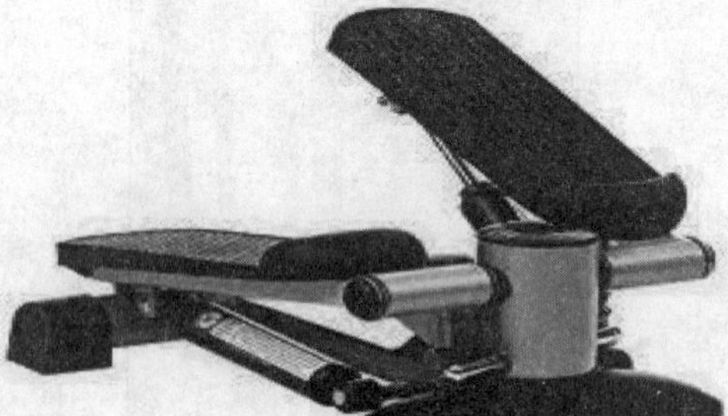

Fig. 8.11: *Stepper*

14. Suspension Apparatus (Guthrie-Smith Frame)

- It mainly used to allow the muscle to contract actively in the gravity eliminated position.
- To improve muscle strength, joint range of motion.
- To decrease pain and muscle spasm. (Fig. 8.12).

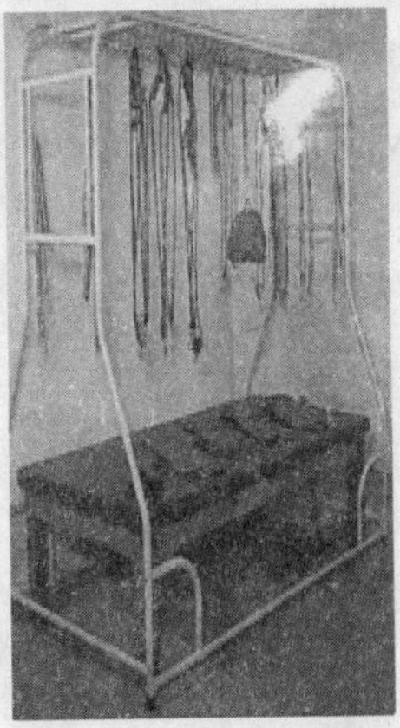

Fig. 8.12: *Suspension apparatus*

15. Walker

- It provide large base of support during walking so it provide more stabilization.
- Help in progressive gait training.
- It improves the confidence of patient during walking. (Fig. 8.13).

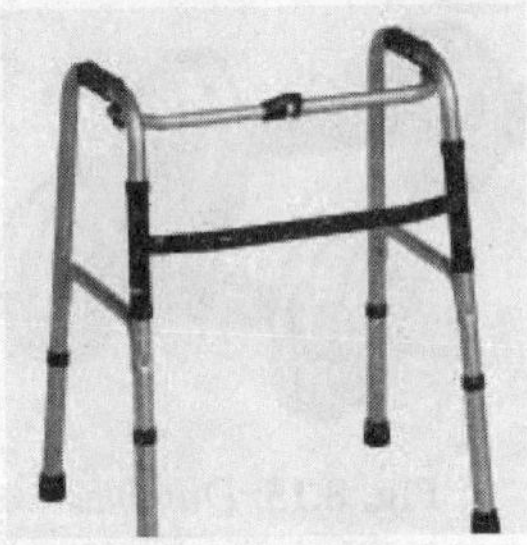

Fig. 8.13: *Walker*

16. Walking sticks- Tripod

- Metal Sticks with three pronged give a more stable support than a stick
- It helps in progressive weight bearing exercises of lower limbs. (Fig. 8.14).

17. Walking sticks- Quadripode

- Metal Sticks with four pronged base give a more stable support.
- It is also used to relief some weight on lower limb. (Fig. 8.14).

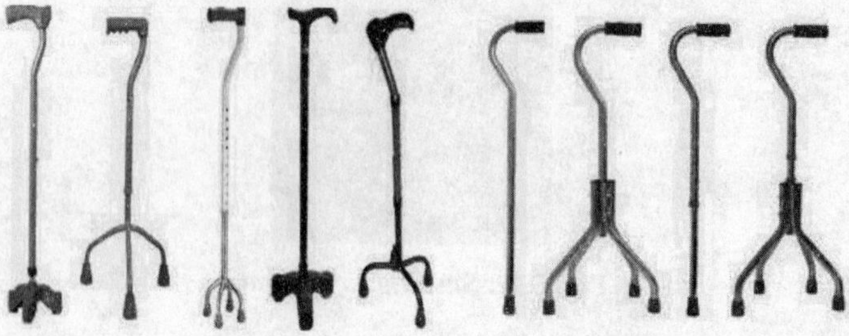

Fig. 8.14: *Walking sticks, Quadruped, Tripods*

18. Dumbles

- It is use to give strengthening of muscle around the elbow joint.
- To improve the muscle bulk. (Fig. 8.15).

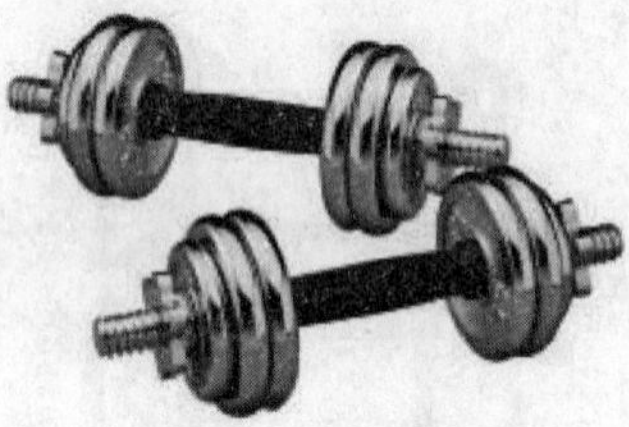

Fig. 8.15: *Dumbles*

19. Elbow Crutches

- They are made of metal and have a metal or plastic forearm band.
- These crutches are particularly suitable for patient with strong arms.
- It transmits the weight of the body. (Fig. 8.16).

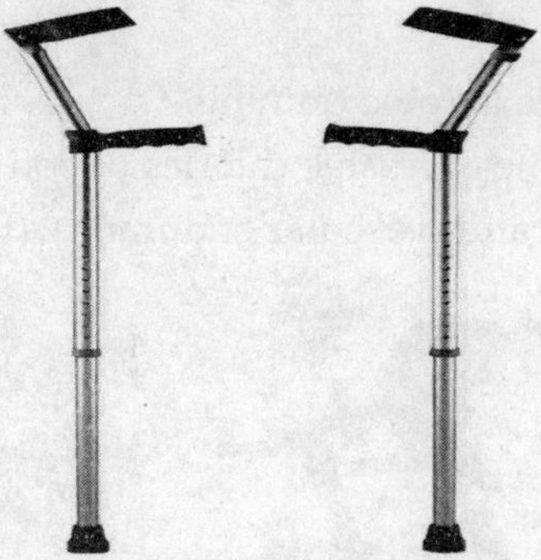

Fig. 8.16: *Elbow crutches*

20. Skin Fold Caliper

- It measured the body fat.
- It measured amount of fat just under the skin at the upper arm, upper back, lower back, stomach and upper thigh.

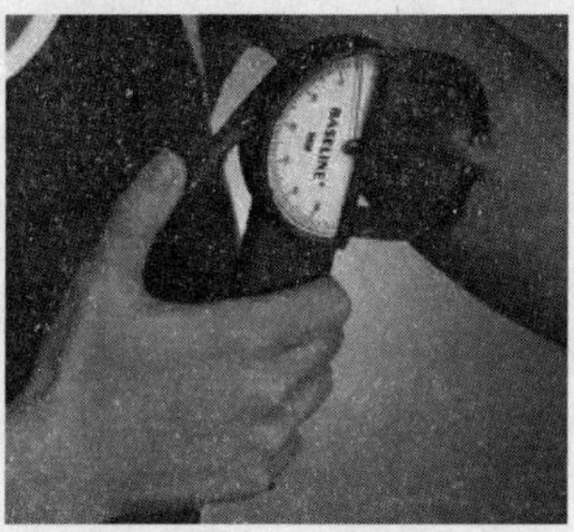

21. Tilt board

- It improves balance.
- Improve neuromuscular reeducation.

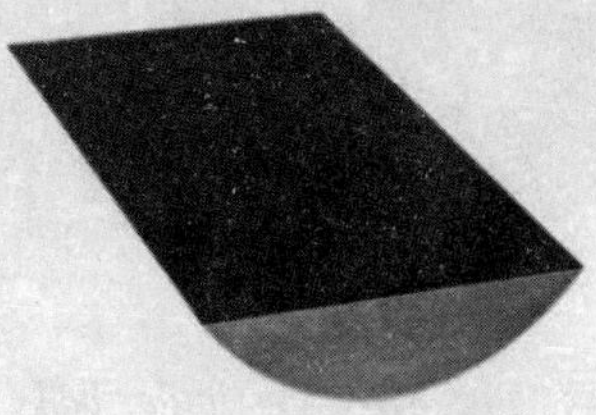

22. Tread Mill

- To provide aerobic training.
- To consume excessive calories of body.
- Improve cardiovascular endurance. (Fig. 8.17).

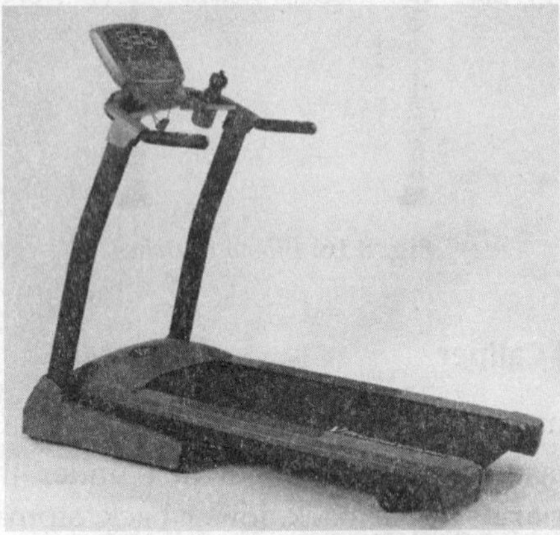

Fig. 8.17: *Tread mill*

23. Vestibular Ball

- It is an inflatable therapy ball designed for gross upper extremity activity balance training activity and total body movement.
- The ball may also be useful in vestibular reflex training. (Fig. 8.18).

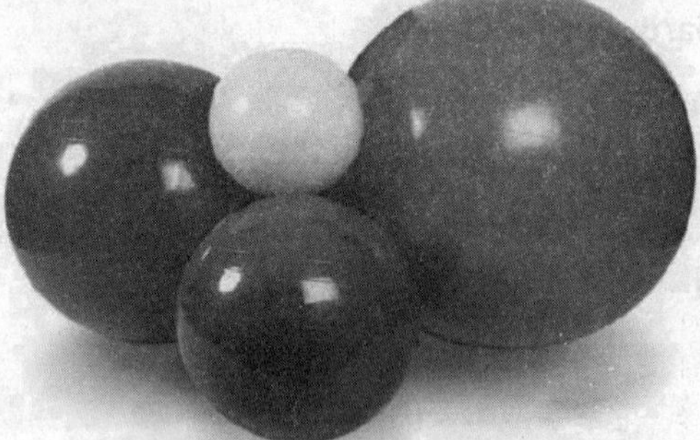

Fig. 8.18: *Vestibular ball*

24. Metal Measuring Tape

- It is used to measure limb length.
- It also used to measure muscle bulk or girth.
- It also used to measure the chest expansion.

25. Arm and Chest Exerciser

- It is used to give resistive exercise of arm and chest.
- It improves the strength of biceps, triceps and pectoralis major muscle. (Fig. 8.19).

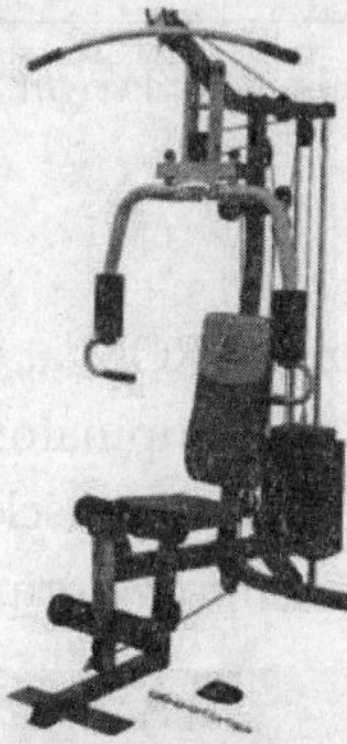

Fig. 8.19: *Arm and chest exerciser*

26. Ball Sorbo Rubber

- This material is used in both compressible and extensible and is useful to provide light resistance for gripping movements of the hand.
- It also improves fine movements of fingers
- It also strengthens the finger and forearm muscles.

27. Weight Cuff

- These cuffs comes in different weight (1Kg, 2Kg, 3Kg, 5Kg etc) and help in resistive exercises.
- To provide resistive exercise of Knee.
- To give isotonic exercises to lower limb. (Fig. 8.20).
- To give exercise for upper limb with weak grip strength.

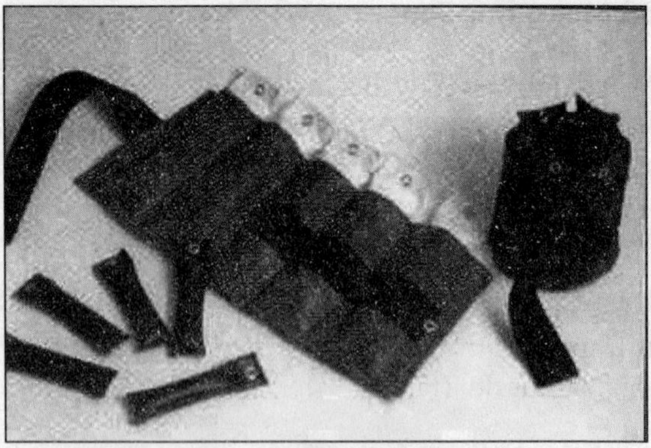

Fig. 8.20: *Weight cuffs*

28. Wrist Rotator

- It is used to increase ROM at wrist joint.
- Resistive exercise of Supinator and pronator.
- Strengthen the forearm muscle.
- It is also used to improve griping. (Fig. 8.21).

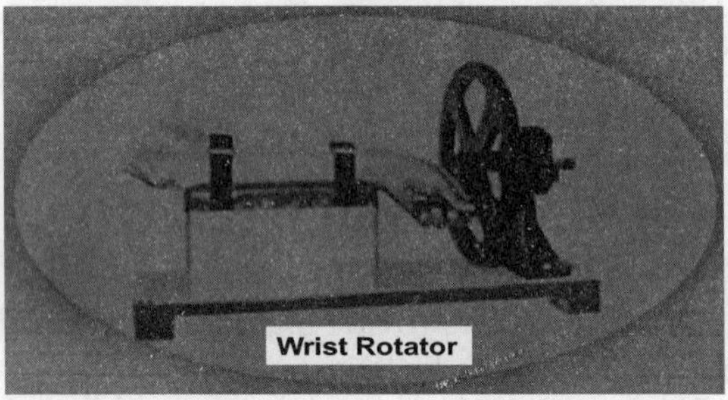

Fig. 8.21: *Wrist rotator*

29. Postural Mirror

- It provides self consciousness during walking or gait training.
- It provides biofeed back to patients during walking.
- It also used for correction of posture. (Fig. 8.22).

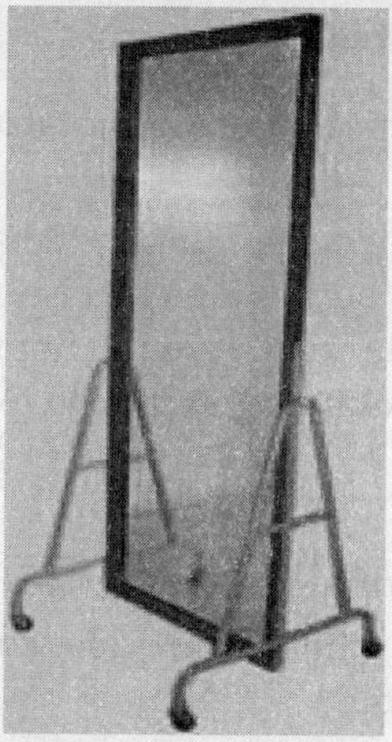

Fig. 8.22: *Postural mirror*

30. Delrome's Shoes

- It is a metallic shoes design for progressive resistive exercises.
- It is useful in assessment and treatment (strengthening) purposes for leg muscles.

31. Latex Tubing

- It is made up of a special type of rubber material for the purpose of a strengthening of upper limb and lower limb muscle.
- It improves the coordination of muscles. (Fig. 8.23).

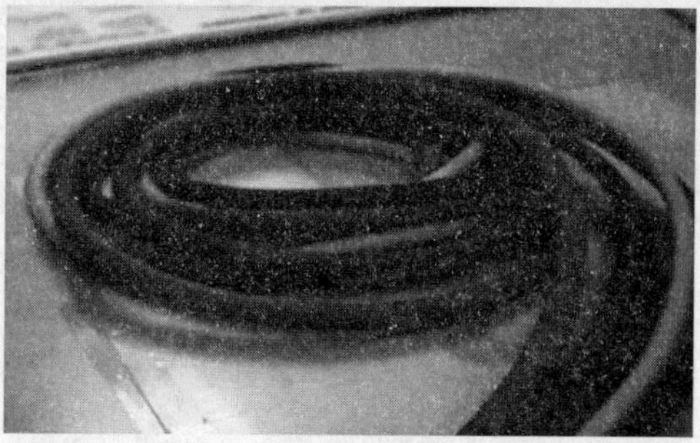

Fig. 8.23: *Latex tubing*

32. Multi Exerciser Table

- It is a special type of therapeutic table for the rehabilitation of upper limb.
- This table includes finger flexion exercise, finger abduction and adduction exercise, wrist deviation, wrist flexion and extension, forearm Supination and Pronation and elbow flexion and extension exercise kit.

33. Peg Boards

- It is made up of wooden material.
- It is simply a square board like structure with different shapes of holes.
- It improves coordination for neurological patients. (Fig. 8.24).

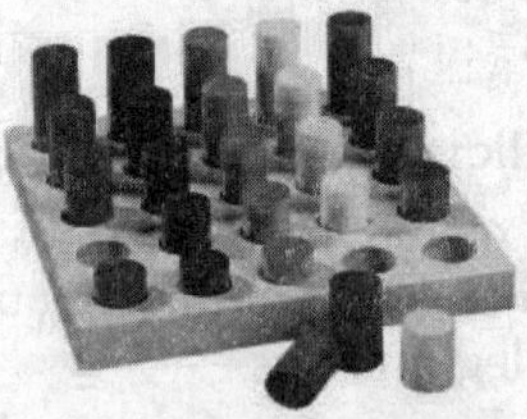

Fig. 8.24: *Peg boards*

34. Rowing Machine

- It is helpful in strengthening of quadriceps muscle.
- Improves passive range of motion for lower limb. (Fig. 8.25).

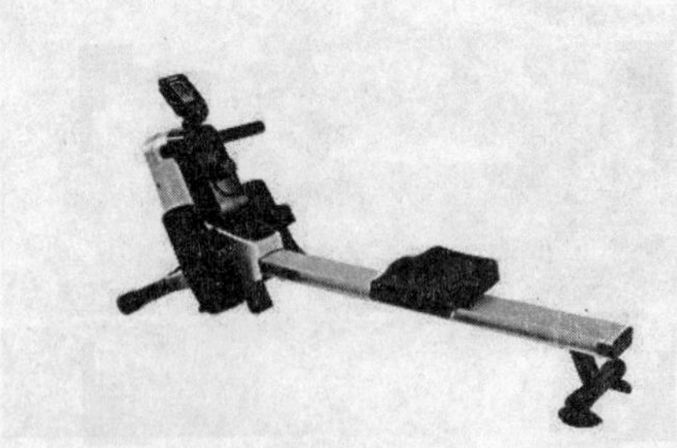

Fig. 8.25: *Rowing machine*

35. Wall Bar

- It just likes a wooden stand on the wall.
- It is helpful in improved balance and confidence to the neurological patient. (Fig. 8.26).

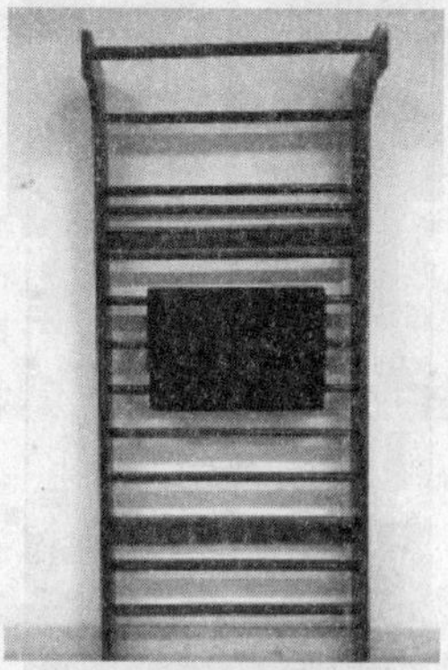

Fig. 8.26: *Wall bar*

36. Peak Flow Meter

- It measures the force of expiration for the cardiovascular patient.
- It improves the strength of expiratory muscles. (Fig. 8.27).

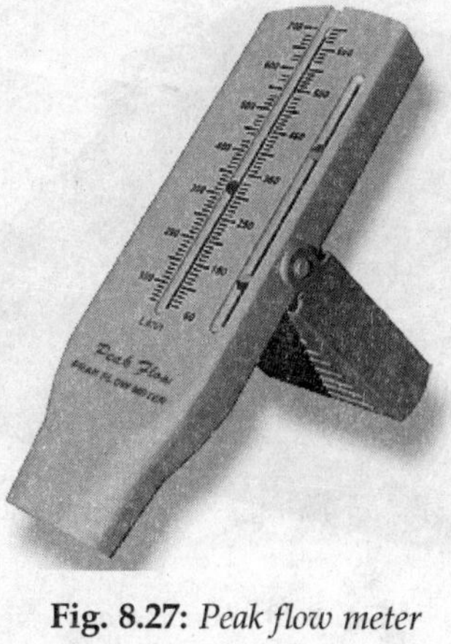

Fig. 8.27: *Peak flow meter*

37. Height Measuring Device

- It is made up of wooden material used for the purpose of measuring height. (Fig. 8.28)

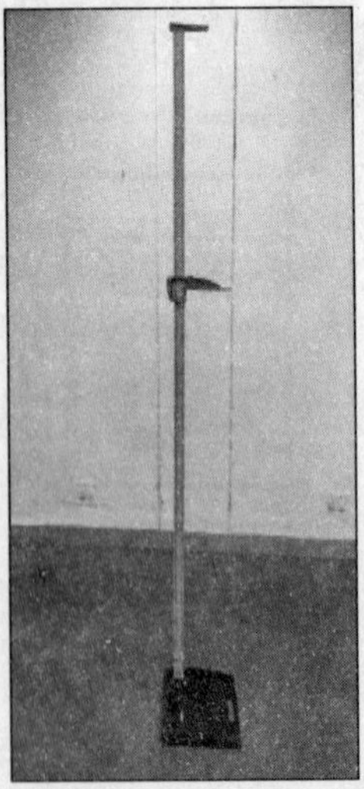

Fig. 8.28: *Height measruing device*

38. Jumbo Mat

- It is a type of exercise mat.
- It is helpful in bed mobility exercises. (Fig. 8.29).

Fig. 8.29: *Jumbo mat*

39. Medicine ball

- Its shape and weight varies according to the requirement.
- It is helpful in coordination and strengthening of upper limb as well as lower limb. (Fig. 8.30).

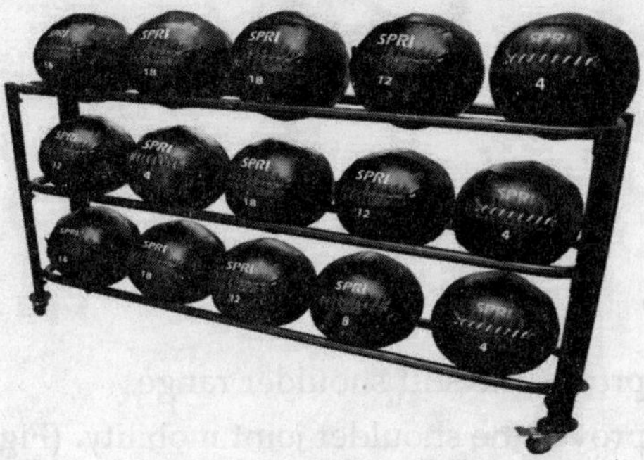

Fig. 8.30: *Medicine ball*

40. Supination and Pronation Exerciser

- Exercises perform at Radioulnar joint.
- It help in improving range of motion at Radioulnar joint. (Fig. 8.31).

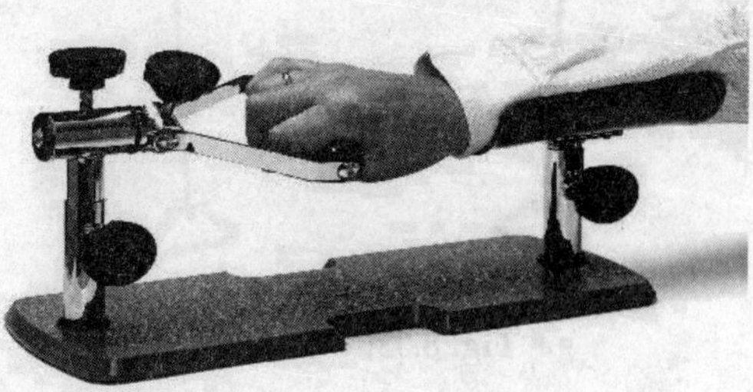

Fig. 8.31: *Supination and pronation exerciser*

41. Quadriceps Table

- It strengthen the leg extensor muscle i.e. quadriceps muscle. (Fig. 8.32).

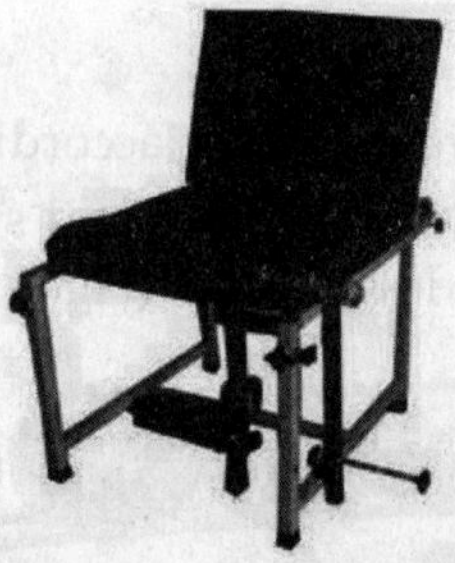

Fig. 8.32: *Quadriceps Table*

42. T- pulley

- It improves the stiff shoulder range.
- It improves the shoulder joint mobility. (Fig. 8.33).

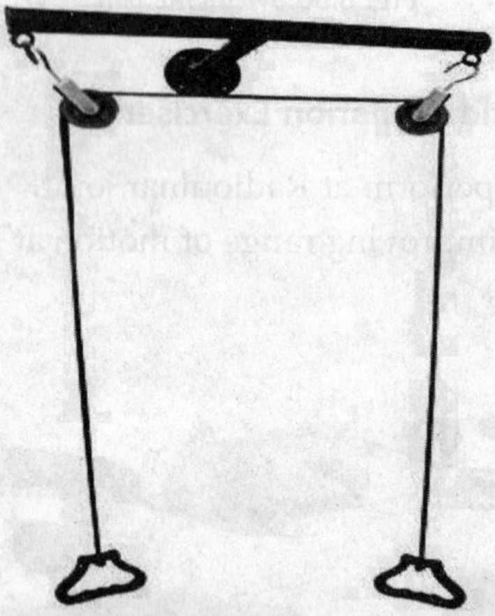

Fig. 8.33: *T- pulley*

43. Pedo Cycle

- It improves the stiff ankle joint range.
- It improves the ankle joint mobility. (Fig. 8.34)

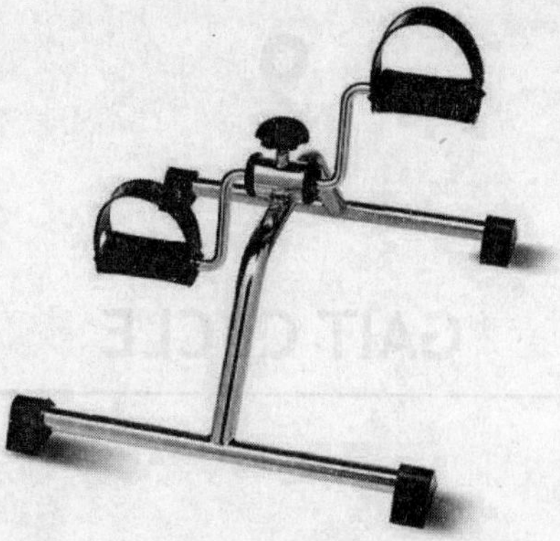

Fig. 8.34: *Pedo cycle*

44. Tilt Table

- It is useful in training the bed ridden patients from lying to standing. (Fig. 8.35).

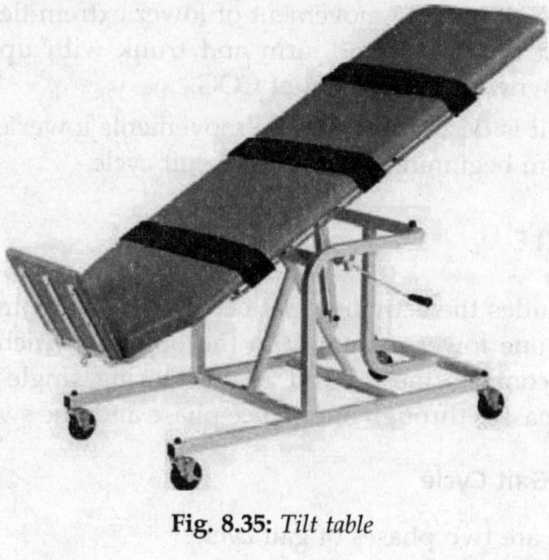

Fig. 8.35: *Tilt table*

9

GAIT CYCLE

GAIT

Gait and human locomotion may be described as a translatory progression as a whole produced by coordinated rotatory movement of body segment.

- It is rhythmic and characterized by alternating propulsive and retropulsive motion of lower extremities.
- The alternative movement of lower extremities, support and carry the head, arm and trunk with upward and downward movement of COG.
- Gait is described by using movements lower extremities from beginning to the end of gait cycle.

GAIT CYCLE

It includes the activities that occur from the point of initial contact of one lower extremity to the point at which the same extremity contacts the ground again. During single gait cycle each limb passes through one stance phase and one swing phase.

Phases of Gait Cycle

There are two phases of gait cycle:

1. Stance phase
2. Swing phase

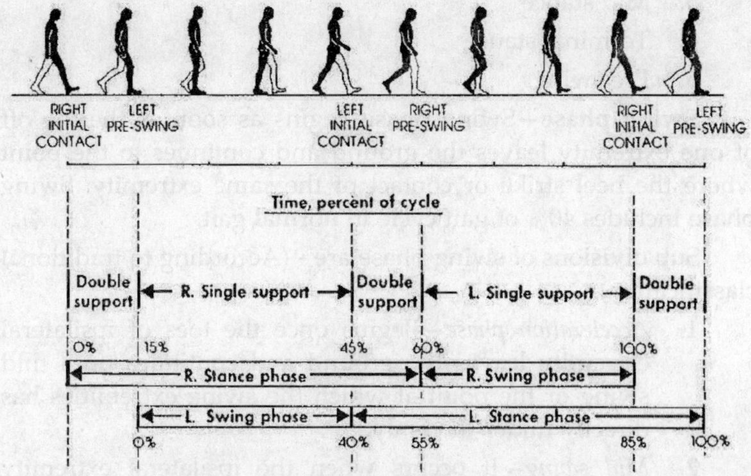

Fig. 9.1: *Phases of gait cycle*

Stance phase—Stance phase begins at the instant that heel of one leading extremity contact the ground and continues only as long as same position of foot is in contact with the ground. It ends when the toe of same foot leaves the ground. Stance phase includes 60 % duration of the gait cycle in a normal gait.

Sub divisions of Stance phase are – (According to traditional classification)

1. *Heel strike* – Heel strike refers to the instant at which the heel of the leading extremities strikes the ground.
2. *Foot flat* – It occurs immediately after heel strike & is the point which the foot fully contact the ground.
3. *Mid stance* – This is a point at which the body weight is directly supporting over the lower extremities.
4. *Heel off* – The point following midstance at which time, heal of the reference extremity leaves the ground.
5. *Toe off* – The point following heal off when only the toe of the reference extremity is in contact with the ground.

Subdivisions of stance phase are - (According to RLA classification)

1. Initial contact
2. Loading response

3. Mid stance
4. Terminal stance
5. Pre swing

Swing phase—Swing phase begins as soon as the toe off of one extremity leaves the ground and continues to the point where the heel strike or contact of the same extremity. Swing phase includes 40% of gait cycle in normal gait.

Sub divisions of swing phase are - (According to traditional classification)-

1. *Acceleration phase*—Begins once the toes of ipsilateral extremity leaves the ground and continues until mid swing or the point at which the swing extremities has directly under the body.
2. *Mid swing*—It occurs when the ipsilateral extremity passes directly beneath the body.
3. *Decceleration phase*—It occurs after mid swing when the tibia passes beyond the perpendicular and knee is standing in preparation for heel strike.

Subdivisions of swing phase are - (According to RLA classification)

1. Initial swing
2. Mid swing
3. Terminal swing

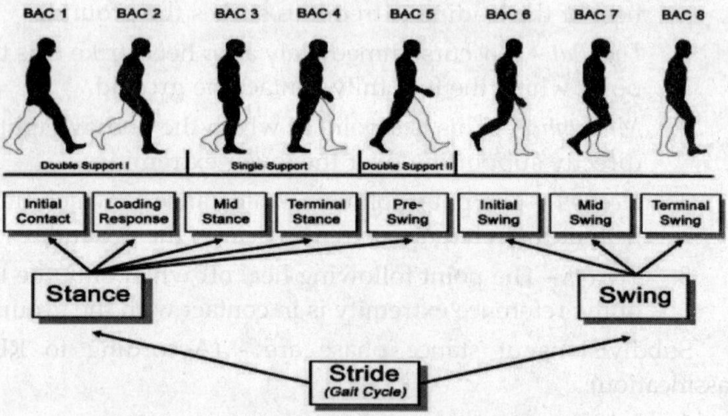

Fig. 9.3: *Subdivisions of stance & swing phase are : (According to RLA classification)*

SOME GENERAL CHARACTERISTICS OF NORMAL GAIT

- Vertical displacement of the center of gravity (COG)
- Lateral displacement of the center of gravity (COG)
- Width of the walking base
- Horizontal dip of the pelvis
- Flexion of knee during stance phase
- Cadence
- Duration of Stance phase is 60% of the cycle
- Duration of Swing phase is 40% of the cycle
- Duration of Double support 22% of the cycle

Vertical Displacement of COG

- The highest point occurs when the supporting limb is in the middle of stance phase.
- The lowest point occurs at the time of durable support when both feet are in contact with the ground.
- The total displacement in an adult is maximum 50 mm.

Lateral Displacement of COG

- The weight is transverse from one leg to other there is shift of pelvis and trunk to the weight bearing side.
- The amount of side to side displacement is in an adult maximum 50 mm.

Width of the Base

- Two lines are drawn through successive mid points of heel strike of each foot.
- The lateral distance between the lines represents the width of the walking base.
- In the great majority of adult males the width of walking base will be within the range of 50 to 100 mm.

Horizontal Dip of Pelvis

- Horizontal dipping of pelvis occurs at first towards the supporting limb then the other limb.

- Normally flexion of knee during stance phase is maximum 20º Knee Flexion and Cadence is 120 steps / min or 2 steps/ sec. Step length - 10 inch to 25 inch.

Flexion of Knee during Stance Phase

This motion is coordinated with the motion at ankle and hip, and keeps the center of gravity at the same level for sometime as it moves forward.

Cadence

- Cadence is the number of steps taken by a person in per unit time.

$$\text{Cadence} = \frac{\text{Step}}{\text{Unit time}}$$

- In normal gate for normal person Cadence is 120 step/ min or 2 step/sec.

KINEMATICS OF NORMAL GAIT

Stance Phase

	Heel strike	*Foot flat*	*Mid stance*	*Heel off*	*Toe off*
MTP	0º	0º	0º	30º	60º Flexion
Ankle Joint	0º	15º Planter flexion	5º Dorsi flexion	0º	20º Plantar flexion
Knee Joint	0º	15º Flexion	5º flexion	0º	35º Flexion
Hip Joint	35º Flexion	25º Flexion	0º	10º Extension	0º

Swing Phase

	Acceleration Phase	*Mid Swing Phase*	*Deceleration Phase*
Ankle Joint	10º Plantar Flexion	0º	0º
Knee Joint	60º Flexion	30º Flexion	0º
Hip Joint	20º Flexion	30º Flexion	30º Flexion

FREQUENTLY USED TERMS

Double support: Total duration of double support is 22% of duration of one gait cycle by both lower extremities. During double support both lower extremities are in contact with the ground at the same time. Absence of double support period distinguishes running from walking.

Stride length: The distance measured by the point of heel strike the reference of same extremities.

Stance time: Stance time is the amount of time elapsed during the stance phase of one extremity in a gait cycle.

Single support time: Amount of time that elapses during the period when only one extremity is only supporting surface in a gait cycle.

Double support time: The amount of time elapsed during both fact of the ground during gait cycle.

Step length: Step length is the linear distance between toes successive points of contact of opposite extremities. It is measured from heel strike from one extremity to heel of opposite extremity.

Width of base support: It is found by measuring of the linear distance between the mid point of heel strike of the foot at the same point on other foot.

Degree of toe out: The angle formed by each foot line of progression and the line of intercepting the centre of heels to the second toe. It is measured by the angle of foot placement the angle is 7° in male at free street walking and in female 4°.

Swing time: Duration of time during gait, when the reference limb is in air.

ABNORMAL GAIT/ PATHOLOGICAL GAIT/ CLINICAL GAIT

The gait which deviates from normal is called abnormal gait. It is also known as pathological gait. Various types of abnormal gait are give below:

Circumductory Gait

This gait is characterized by the action of circumduction at the affected joint instead of flexion of hip joint abducted and externally rotated thus the circumductory gait also happen because increase in the apparent length of the limb. It is also seen in case of planter flexed foot. e.g. Hemiplegic gait. (Fig. 9.4).

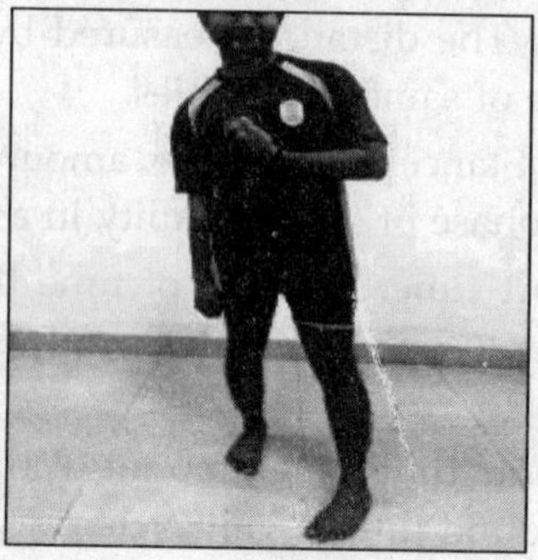

Fig. 9.4: *Circumductory Gait*

Scissor Gait

This gait is characterized by crossing the leg because both adductors of hip joint become hypertonic or contracture of the both adductor of hip joint. e.g. – C.P. Child (Cerebral Palsy Child). (Fig, 9.5).

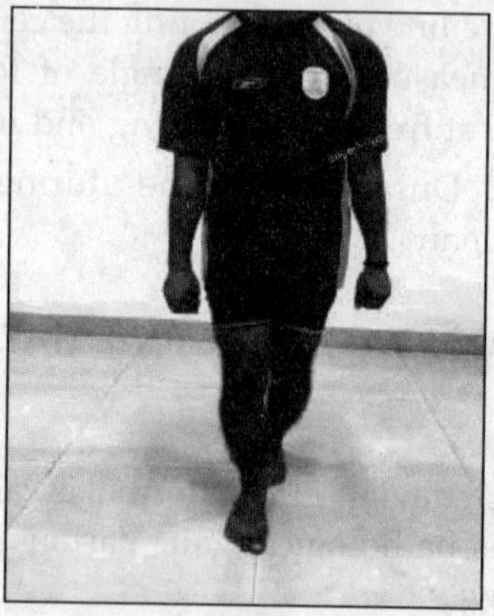

Fig. 9.5: *Scissor Gait*

Antalgic Gait

It is possible in painful lower limbs. Person spends less time on the stance phase. e.g. - Painful limb.

Shuffling Gait

It is also known as festinating gait. The gait is characterized by short stride means stride length is shorter than the normal. The speed of walking is quicker than the normal this is because of the rigidity of the muscle. Patient is unable to stop voluntary rigidity. e.g. – Parkinson's disease. (Fig, 9.6).

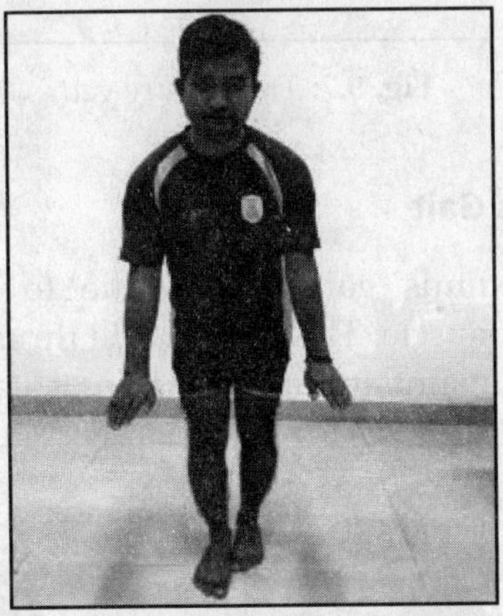

Fig. 9.6: *Shuffling gait*

Unsteady Gait

This gait is characterized by unsteadiness of the involuntary movement of the both limbs and trunk. The unsteadiness in walking with speed. e.g. – Athetoid type of C.P.

Tredlenburg Gait

It is known as Gluteus medius gait this is because of weakness of gluteus medius muscle .Occur in an unstable hip due to congenital dislocation of hip which leads to gluteus medius weakness. Any pathological conditions or weakness in gluteus medius on one side causes a contralateral pelvic drop. (Fig, 9.7).

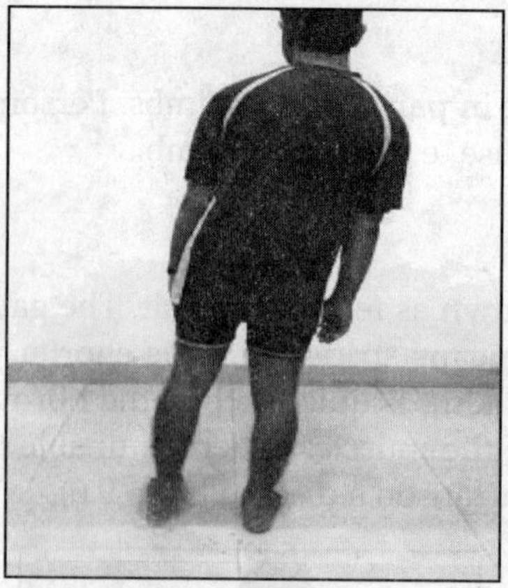

Fig. 9.7: *Tredlenburg gait*

Gluteus Maximus Gait

Gluteus maximus gait occurs due to the weakness of gluteus maximus muscle. The patient will thrust thorax posterior at initial stance to maintain hip extension of stance leg. (Fig, 9.8).

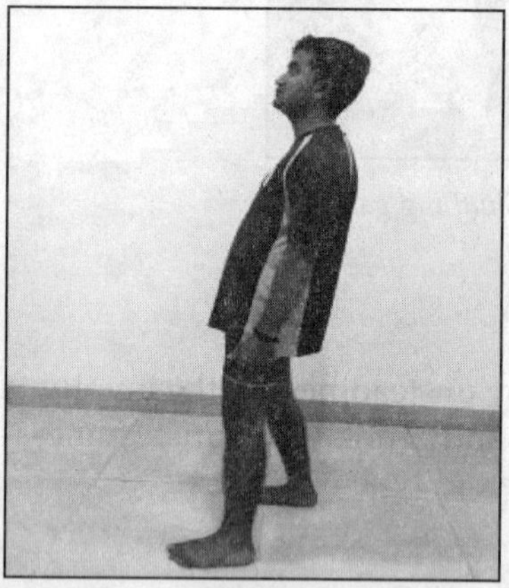

Fig. 9.8: *Gluteus maximus gait*

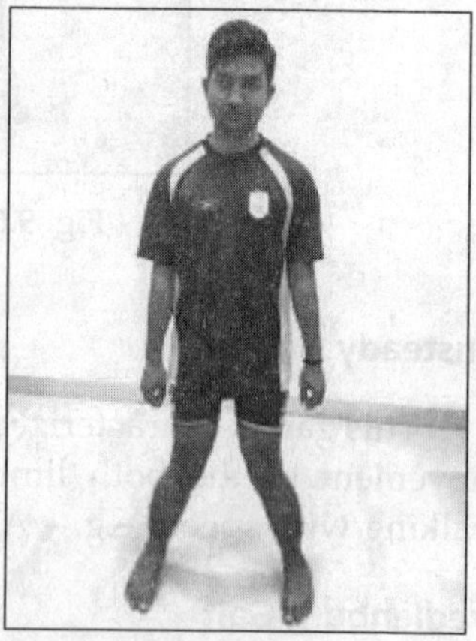

Fig. 9.8 A: *Waddling gait*

Waddling Gait

It is characterized by waddle is caused by adductor muscle weakness. In this condition the base of support increases. Perhaps a person can walk in weakness of lower limb musculature. e.g. – Poliomyelitis.

Ataxic Gait

Ataxic gait is due to poor sensation or lack of muscles co – ordination. The gait of individual limb which include lurch or stagger and movement are exaggerated. e.g. cerebral Ataxia. The resulting gait is irregular and waving. (Fig, 9.9).

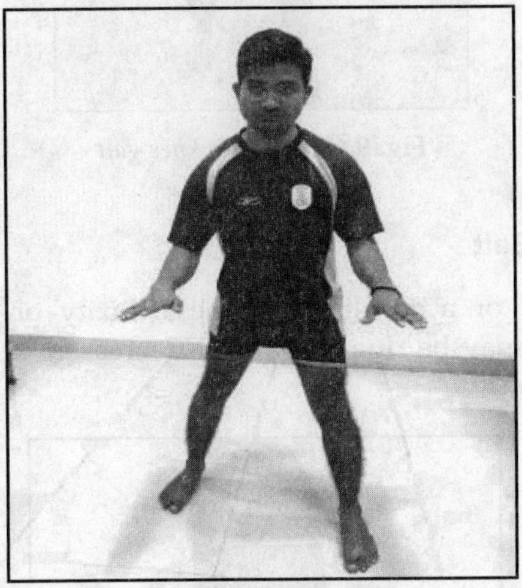

Fig. 9.9: *Ataxic gait*

Hysterical Gait

It seen in patient of Psychological Disorder. This patient feet or foot describes half circles with each step. e.g. – Typical Hysterical gait.

Kinesia Paradise

In this one can run easily or better than walking.

Hand to Knee Gait

This is due to weakness in quadriceps femoris. It is characterized by supporting the knee with hand in order to prevent buckling of knee during walking. (Fig, 9.10).

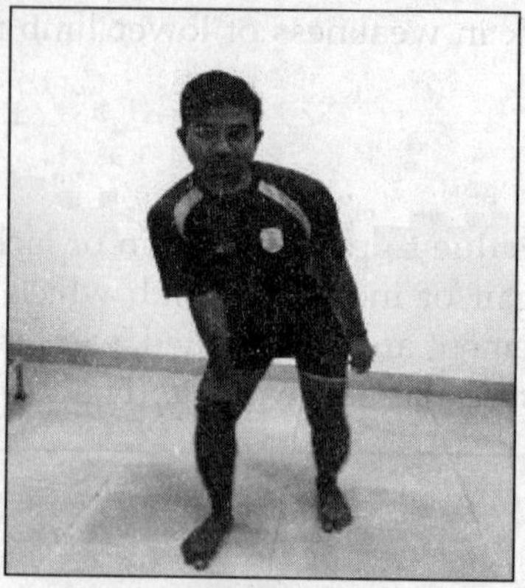

Fig. 9.10: *Hand to knee gait*

Anthrogenic Gait

It occurs or a result of stiffness, laxity or deformity of joint all it. It may be due to painful decreased ROM free joint. (Fig. 9.11).

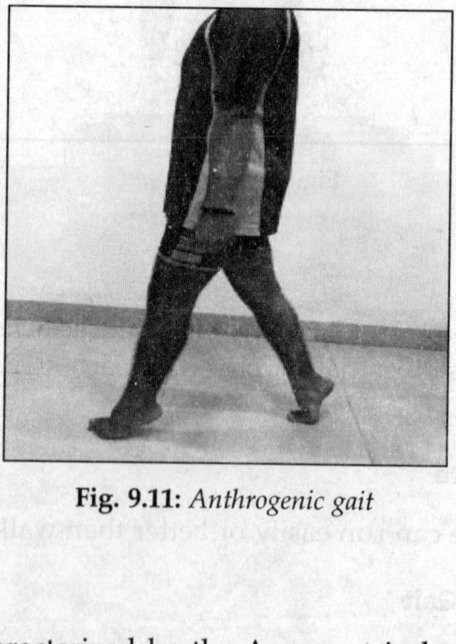

Fig. 9.11: *Anthrogenic gait*

Limping Gait

This is characterized by the Asymmetrical gait. The swing phase gets increase and stance phase gets decreased on the affected side.

High Steppage Gait

This is because of the weakness of dorsiflexors of the ankle joint. Clearly seen in foot drop condition. Person walking with high swing limb to clear the ground. (Fig. 9.12).

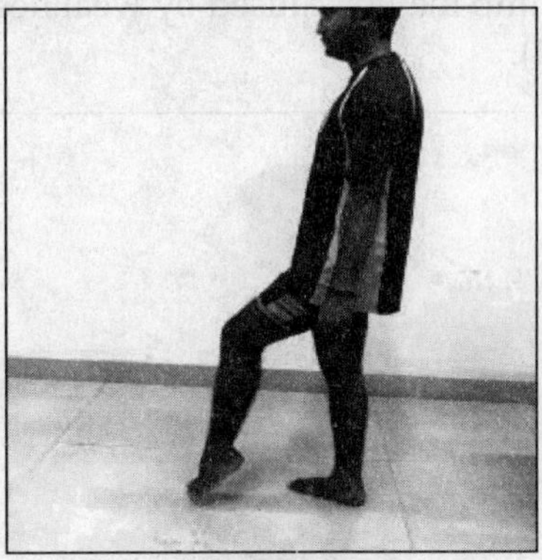

Fig. 9.12: *High steppage gait*

Short Leg Gait

If one leg is shorter than the other or there is deformity in one of the bones of the leg. The patient will demonstrate lateral shift to the affected side and the pelvic tilt downwards on the affected side. (Fig. 9.13).

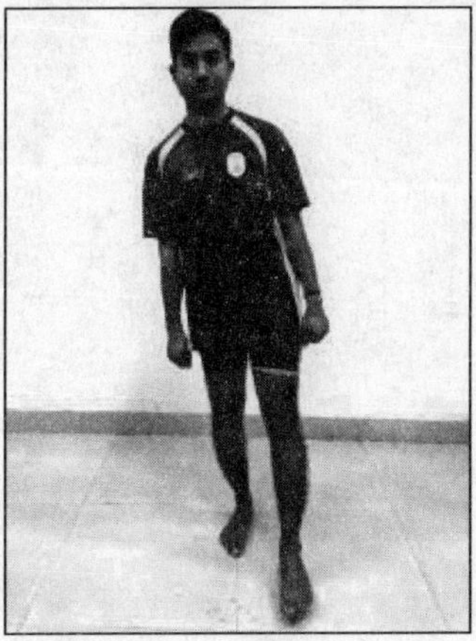

Fig. 9.13: *Short leg gait*

Psoatic Limb

It is seen in patients with Leg – Calve – Perthes disease. The patient demonstrates the difficulty in swing through, and the limp may be accompanied by exaggerated trunk and pelvic movement. The limp may be caused by weakness of Psoas major muscle. (Fig. 9.14).

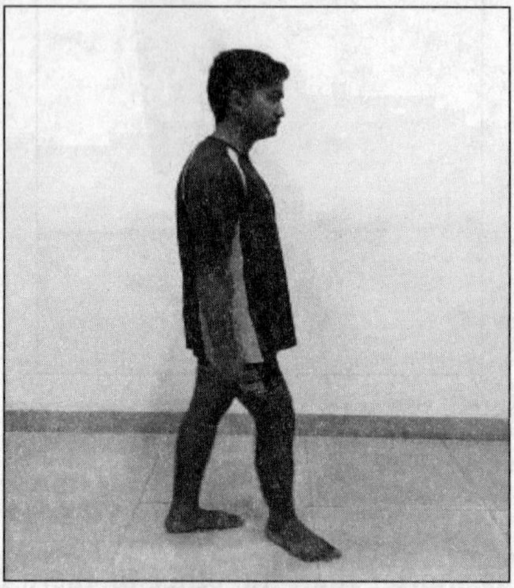

Fig. 9.14: *Psoatic Limb*

NOTE : The gait pattern of a person reflects occupation, body structure healthy status, personality and other physical and psychological background.

10

MASSAGE OR SOFT TISSUE MANIPULATION (S.T.M.)

INTRODUCTION

Massage or S.T.M. is a procedure in which soft tissue mobilization is done with the help of hands or electrical equipment known as massager (Fig. 10.1). It is for curative purpose or palliative purpose (Palliative – Apparent recovery but not real). Before massage following points should be considered by the therapist –

- Full knowledge of anatomy and physiology
- Hands should be clean, warm
- Finger nail should be cut, rings and wrist watch should be removed.
- Purposeful attitude
- Healthy, clean and airy atmosphere

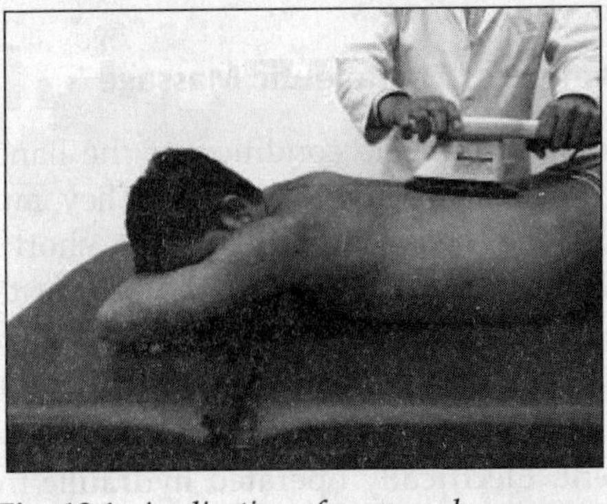

Fig: 10.1: *Application of massage by massager*

COMPONENT CONSIDERED AMONG STM

Direction of Movement

- Centripetal or centrifugal direction [Proximal to distal] may be follow, depending upon the purpose.
- This is for the soothing effect [i.e. false feeling of relaxation only to the mental effect].
- In case of belly to be manipulated, direction should be along the muscle fiber.
- Massage when proceed distal to proximal direction help to maintain venous return as well as lymph return in some massage techniques such as deep friction and connective tissue massage (CTM).

Pressure

- It should be firm and deep but should not be forceful.
- Soothing and warming effect by low pressure.
- For adhesions and contractures, pressure should be deep and firm.

Rate and Rhythm

For simulating quick and strong 15 strokes/minute and rate 1-2 inch/second, slow and rhythmic.

Medium

Medium should be oily or talcum powder or cream should be applied to reduce friction between the therapist hand and patient skin.

Basic Requirement of Therapeutic Massage

Hand Preparation: The condition of the hand is extremely important to both therapist and patient. They must be cleaned and groomed. The nails should be kept short and the tips rounded, and they should not injure the patient through any of the massage stroke. **Lubricants:** Powder, Oil and cream are used as lubricant to facilitate movement of the hands over the body tissues.

Equipment: Electrically operated hydraulic treatment table. (Fig: 10.2).

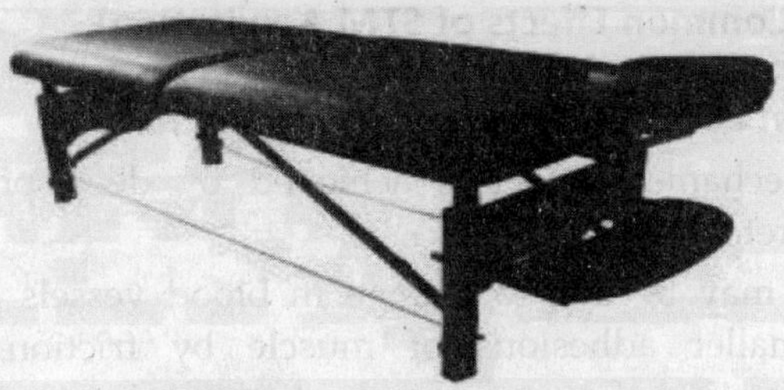

Fig: 10.2: *Massage table*

Position

1. Position should be comfortable, affected part should be well supported within the reach of therapist hand.
2. For the edema and swelling of the limb elevation should be preferred.

Type of Movement

1. Depending upon the Physiotherapist's hand condition and technique type of movement should be decided.
2. Vibration associated with gravity move the secretions from bronchiole to bronchia and to trachea. Secretions from trachea is expelled by coughing.

Indication

- To stimulate circulation
- To increase metabolism
- Nutrition to the part affected
- To increase warmth of the skin.
- To dissolve soft tissue adhesion.
- To decrease swelling.
- To decrease muscle spasm and soothing effect.
- To stretch contracture.
- To attain relaxation.
- To stimulate cough and clear air passages.

EFFECTS (Common Effects of STM Application)

Mechanical effect (Application of external force)

- Mechanical effect is achieved by deep pressure and stretching.
- It may be due to change in blood vessels or to break smaller adhesions of muscle by friction or loosen secretion of mucous by chest percussion.

Physiological effect

- Increase temperature of skin or warmth the skin.
- Increase blood circulation of skin.
- Makes skin softer.
- Increase elasticity of soft tissue.

Circulatory effect

- Deep pressure in flaccid paralysis may increase Blood flow.
- Release of histamine and acetylcholine as a result of vasodilatation of blood vessels so the Blood flow increases.

Effect on lungs

- Percussion with postural drainage may causes secretion of mucous i.e. move in a direction at a time.
- Movement should be continuous while hand is in contact with the skin.

TECHNIQUE

Manipulation are most effectively performance with the hands and are administrated for the purpose of producing effect on the Nervous system, Muscles and respiratory system and local and general circulation of Blood flow and lymph.

(1) Stroking

Stroking movement is performed with the entire palmer surface of one or both hands moving in any direction on the surface of body. Stroking can been given in any direction however the direction should be one i.e. convenient for the operator and comfortable to the patient.

Rate of movement

- Stroking may be slow or fast.
- If performed slowly it tends to be relaxing, if performed quickly it has more stimulating effect on the tissue.

Depth and pressure

- Light pressure for superficial structures and greater pressure for deep structures should be performed.
- Superficial stroking is usually slow and gentle but firm i.e. enough for the patient who should be conscious for passage of the hand throughout the movement.
- Deep stroking tends to stimulate the circulation of deep muscle tissue.
- It is generally given in the direction of venous and lymph flow.

Effect of stroking

- Significant relaxation producing a sedative effect may help relieving pain and muscle spasm (Pain gate mechanism).
- Stimulation may cause dilatation of arteries in deeper tissue and in superficial structure.
- Promotes relaxation and induces sleep in person with insomnia.

Therapeutic uses of stroking

- General and Local relaxation.
- Relieves muscle spasm, indirectly pain may be relieved.

Contraindication

- Large open area
- Gross edema
- Varicosities
- Hyperthermia
- Extremely hairy area [head, maxilla, genital organ]

(2) Effleurage

It is a slow striking movement performed with increasing pressure in the direction of return of blood and lymph flow [Distal to proximal]. Hence must be relaxed and molded accurately to the shape of the part being treated. The stroke should be smooth and rhythmic and must be directed towards the group of lymph gland following the courses of superficial veins and lymphatics.

- Initial effleurage. (Fig: 10.3A)
- End position of effleurage. (Fig: 10.3B)
- Return stroke or second stroke. (Fig: 10.3C)

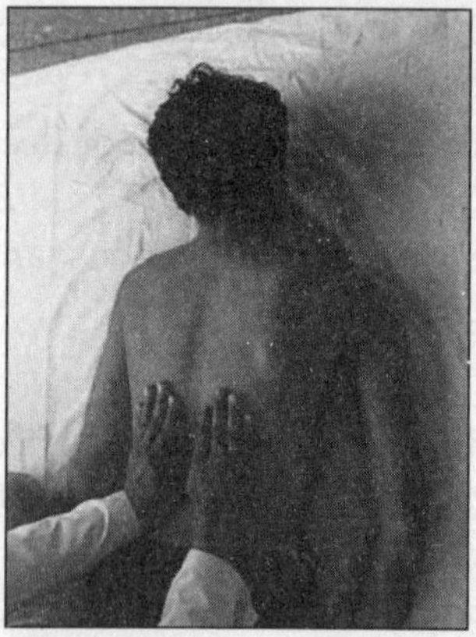

Fig: 10.3A: *Initial effleurage*

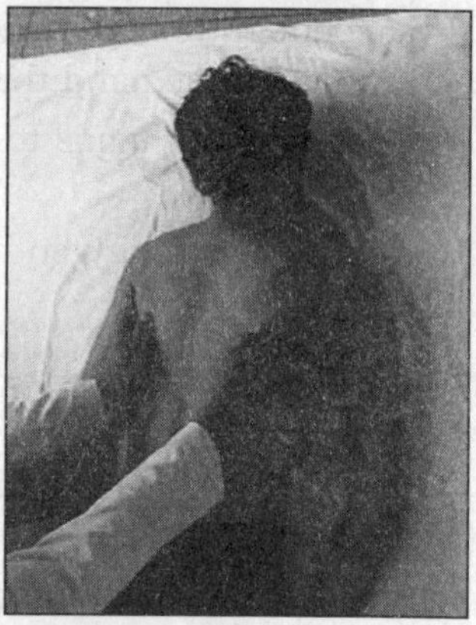

Fig: 10.3B: *End position of effleurage*

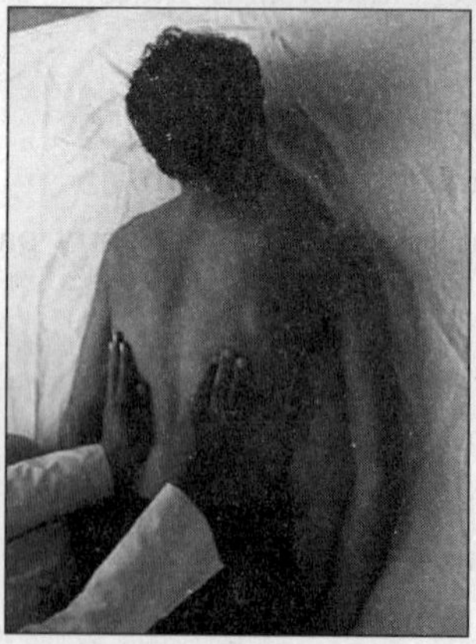

Fig: 10.3C: *Return stroke or second stroke*

RATE OF MOVEMENT: 6-7 INCH/ SECOND

Pressure

Pressure should be gradually increased so that the venous blood and lymph are pushed through the veins and lymph channels. There should be definite pause at the end of each stroke at or near the lymph gland.

Effect of Effleurage

Mechanical effect

- By mechanical pressure the flow of blood in superficial veins is moved towards the heart.
- Help in elimination of waste product.
- Stimulate circulation.
- Mobility of superficial soft tissue is increased.
- Increased circulation lead to improved healing process.

Therapeutic effect

- General and Local relaxation.
- Relief muscle spasm indirectly pain may be relieved.

Contraindication

- Large open area
- Varicosities
- Gross oedema
- Hyperthermia
- Extremely hairy area.

(3) Petressage (Pressure-manipulation)

It is characterized by firm pressure applied to the tissue. Its aims to mobilize the deep muscle tissue, skin or subcutaneous tissue. It is of four types:-

1. **Kneading**–Kneading is performed by thumb, manipulation in which muscle and subcutaneous tissue are alternately compressed and released, movement takes place in circular motion. During the pressure phase of each stroke, the skin and hands are moved

together [By both or unilateral thumbs] Kneading help to mobilize other deep tissue and muscle fiber. It also helps to mobilize chronic swelling specialty when swelling has become organized. Various techniques adapted during kneading-

(i) Compression kneading
(ii) Squeeze kneading
(iii) Finger pad kneading
(iv) Reinforce kneading (Fig. 10.4)
(v) Knuckle kneading (Fig. 10.5)
(vi) Thumb pad kneading (Fig.10.6)

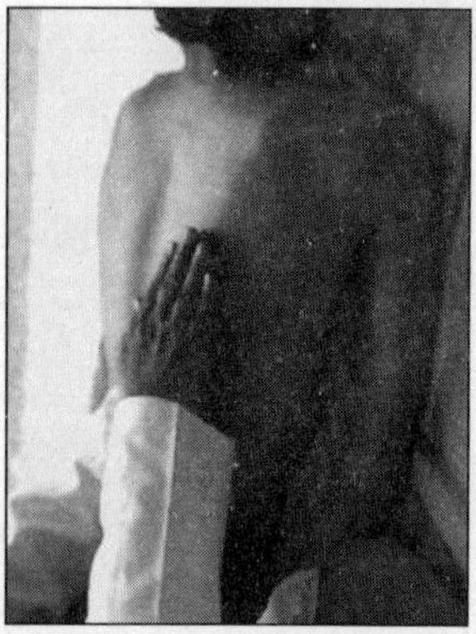

Fig: 10.4: *Reinforce kneading*

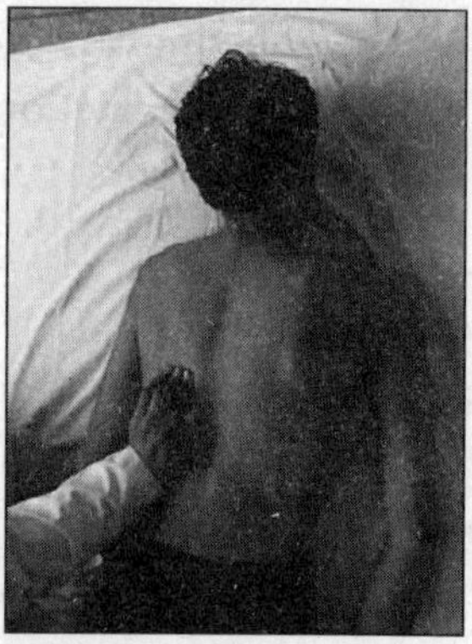

Fig: 10.5: *Knuckle kneading*

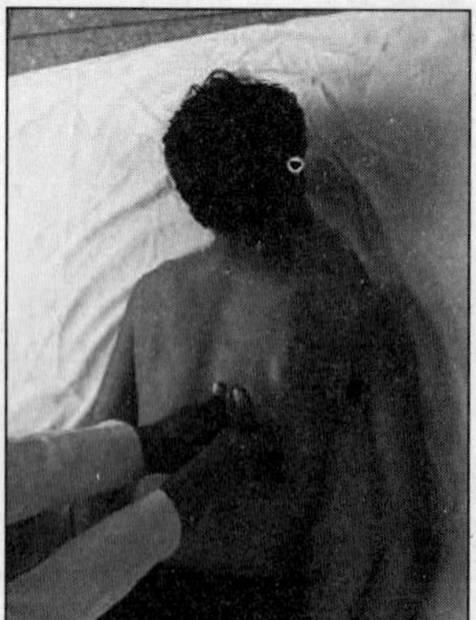

Fig: 10.6: *Thumb pad kneading*

2. **Picking up**—One or more muscles are grasped, lifted away from under lying tissues, squeezed and released. They are grasped and released in a circular manner. (Fig. 10.7).

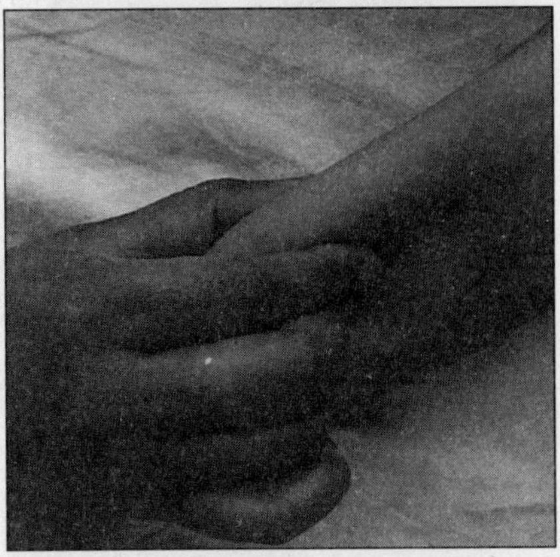

Fig: 10.7: *Picking up*

3. **Wringing**—It is a manipulation in which tissues are lifted with both hands and compressed alternatively between finger and thumb of opposite hand. Speed must be about 4-6 inches/second for large muscle. (Fig. 10.8)

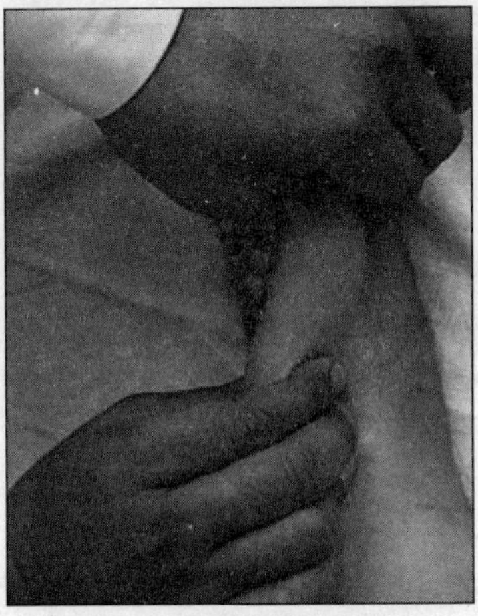

Fig: 10.8: *Wringing*

4. **Skin rolling** – In skin rolling the skin and subcutaneous tissue are rolled over the deeper structures. It is used mainly for the improving circulation. (Fig. 10.9).

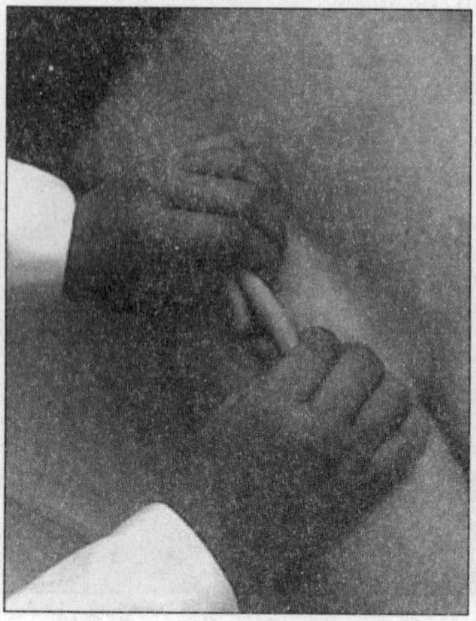

Fig: 10.9: *Skin rolling*

Effects of Petressage

Physiological effect

- Flow of lymph is stimulated by some mechanical pressure.
- Increased blood supply.
- Slow rhythmic petressage relaxes muscles and reduces pain.
- It mobilizes by manipulation and that promotes elasticity.

Therapeutic effect

- Mobilize muscle contracture.
- Mobilizes the skin and subcutaneous tissue.
- Resolve pain and muscle fatigue.

Contraindication

- Deep kneading to acute muscle tear.
- Around acutely inflamed joint.
- Skin disease e.g. - dermatitis, infection.

- Hyper or hypotonic limb.
- Malignant disease or bacterial infection.

(4) Tapotemant

Tapotemant is also known as Percussion Manipulation. Hand working alternatively and wrist are kept flexible so that the movements are light spinning and stimulating. It is of four types-

1. **Hacking**—Hacking is a single or double handed stroke in which lateral edge and dorsal surface of the finger strike skin surface in rapid succession, mainly through the V, IV and III finger (Fig. 10.10). This creates strong stimulating effect. Stimulating basically the skin and subcutaneous tissue and muscle tissue.

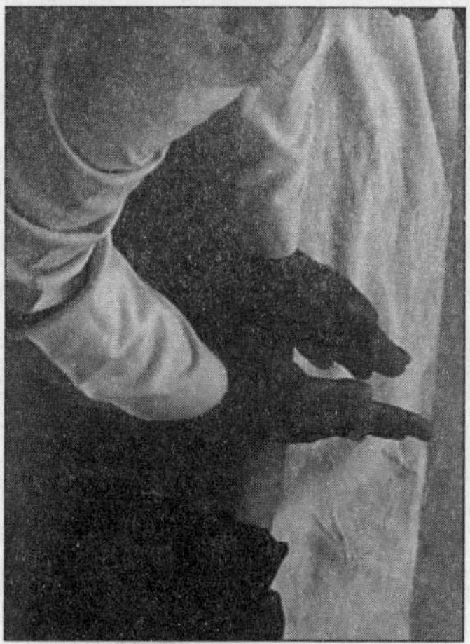

Fig. 10.10: *Hacking*

2. **Clapping**—Clapping is single or two handed stroke in which cupped hand strike on the skin surface rapidly (Fig. 10.11). Compressing the air and causing the vibration wave to penetrate the tissue. Effect- Clapping is designed to stimulate tissue by direct method. It may be performed on the lung tissues, mechanical effect helps to loosen the secretions.

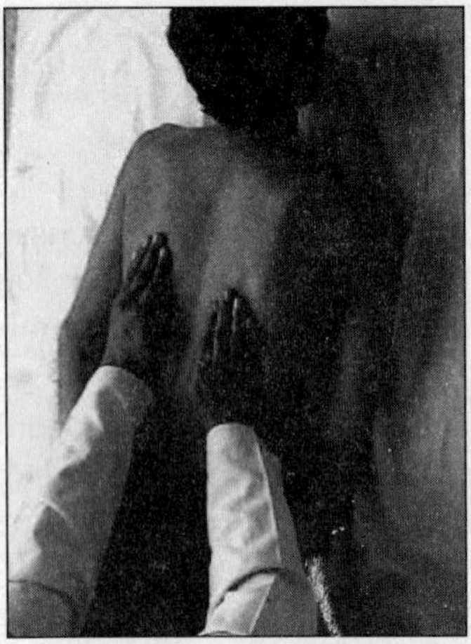

Fig. 10.11: *Clapping*

3. **Beating**–Beating is designed to stimulate the tissue by direct mechanical action. Basically to the sacrum region it gives very effective stimulating effect through the distal phalanx in the beating process. Beating is a single or two handed stroke in which loosely clinched fist strike the part so that dorsal aspect of middle phalanx and distal phalanx of the finger make contact with the patient skin. (Fig. 10.12).

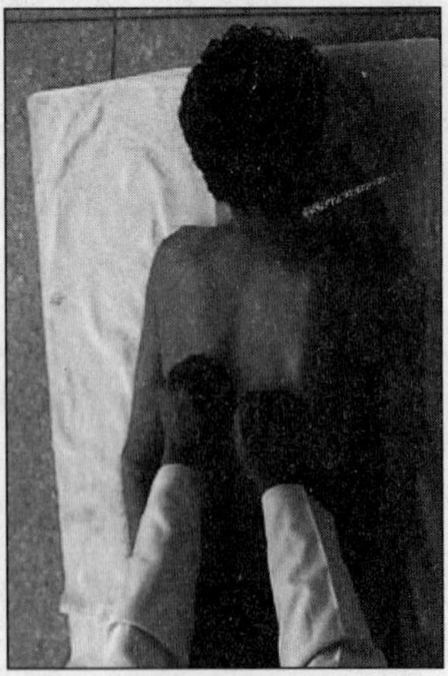

Fig. 10.12: *Beating*

4. **Pounding**–Pounding is a movement in which the ulnar border of hand with loosely clinched fist and rapid successive strike are given to the part to be treated. It is somewhat deeper than the hacking. Purpose is same like hacking but depth is greater than the hacking. (Fig. 10.13)

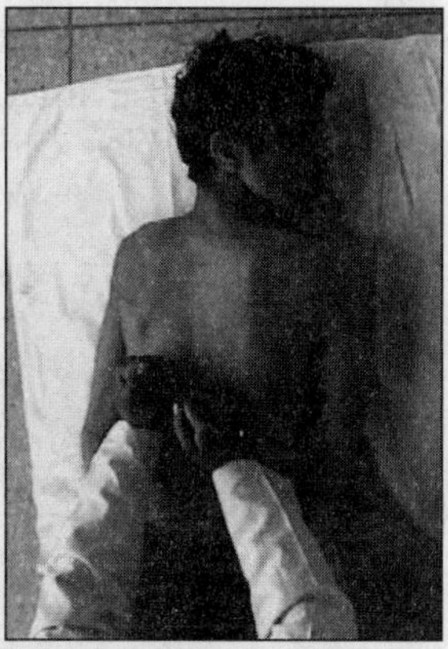

Fig. 10.13: *Pounding*

Effect of Tapotemant

Mechanical effect

It is given over the thorax so that adherent mucous can be loosened and moved along the respiratory tract. This is suitable in the postural drainage position (Half lying).

Reflex effect

Stimulation of vasomotor nerve, hacking ever the spinal muscle may induce general sernse of warmth, by stimulation of sensory branch of posterior primary rami. Tapotemant over the muscle fiber produces stretching effect that facilitates muscle contraction by reflex stimulation of sensory nerve ending. It is given for pain relief through spinal mechanism.

Therapeutic effect

- In chest conditions such as chronic fibrosis, bronchectasis.
- General stimulating effect to any part of body.
- To relief neuralgia following complications of trauma and other pathological processes.

Contraindication

- Spasticity [may be increase]
- Bony prominent area

(5) Vibration

Vibration is a single or double handed technique in which the fine shaking movement or tremor is conveyed to the tissue by hands or finger tips. It designed primarily to help loosening the secretion. Vibration over muscles can stimulate a stretch reflex. (Fig. 10.14).

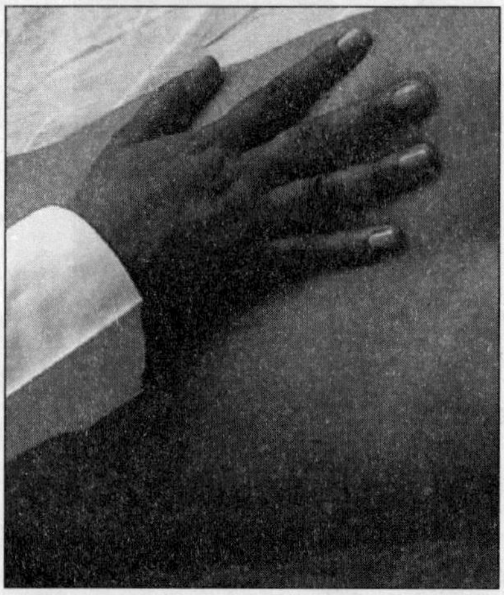

Fig. 10.14: *Vibration*

(6) Shaking

- Shaking is a single or double handed technique in which a rhythmic shaking movement or tremor is conveyed to the tissue by finger tips or hands. (Fig. 10.15).
- Shaking is a stroke designed primarily to assist in the loosening of secretion from the lungs. It is similar to vibration but it usually performed rather than the vibration.
- Shaking is more vigorous stroke than the vibrations and therefore more pressure is applied during actual shaking of the chest.

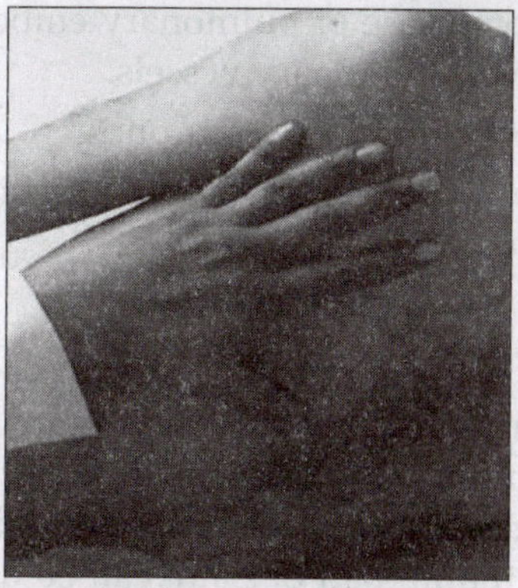

Fig. 10.15: *Shaking with hand*

Effect of Vibration and Shaking

Mechanical effect

- Loosening adherent mucous.
- May help to reduce oedema.
- May applied over stomach and intestine and the manipulation causes movement of gas.

Reflex effect

Vibration applied over nerve may relief pain. This technique may be also used to facilitate the muscle contraction.

Therapeutic effect

- For chronic chest conditions and following chest surgery to loosen mucus.
- Aids expectorant in the respiratory tract.
- Helps in resolving chronic edema for the relief in some cases of neuralgia.

Contraindication of Shaking and Vibration

1. Shaking and vibration may cause obvious damage to the under lying lung tissue if given over the thoracic region.
2. To thorax in case of heart failure specially associated with coronary thrombosis.

3. To thorax in case of pulmonary embolism it may cause blockage of pulmonary vessels.
4. In case of severe hypertension.
5. In case of hyperesthesia. [Hypersensitive]
6. Spasticity

(7) Deep Friction

Deep friction consist of small accurate, localized deeply, penetrating per movement perform in a circular or transverse direction. These deep strokes are fully carried out by the finger tips, through the thumb pad or palm can be used. (Fig. 10.16).

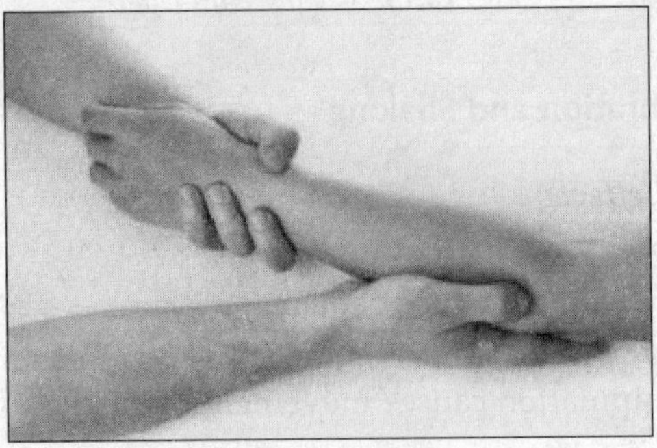

Fig. 10.16: *Deep friction*

Purpose

Deep friction is designed to mobilize tendon, ligament, joint capsule and muscle tissue, particularly chronic adhesion or inflammation.

Effect of Soft Tissue Manipulation [S.T.M.]

Mechanical Effect

- Movement of lymph, blood vessels, lungs secretion, edema, interstitial contents, Hematoma contents (Internal sloughing of blood in vessels).
- Mobilization of muscle fiber, muscle masses, tendon, skin or subcutaneous tissue, scar tissue.
- Adhesions breaking.

Physiological effect

- To increase circulation of blood and lymph.
- Increase flow of nutrients.
- Removal of waste product and metabolites.
- Stimulation of healing process.
- Increase extensibility of connective tissue.
- Pain relief.
- Increase joints movements.
- Facilitation of muscle activity.
- Stimulation of autonomic function.
- Removal of lungs secretion.
- Sexual arousal.
- Promotion of local and general relaxation.

Psychological effect (Palliative effect)

- Physical relaxation
- Relief of tension and anxiety.
- Stimulation of physical activity
- Pain relief
- General feeling of well being.
- Sexual arousal.

Therapeutic effect

- General and local relaxation.
- To relief chronic edema.
- Scar tissue.
- Lesion of tendon, ligament or joint & hematoma.
- Chronic constipation.
- Facilitation movement and prevention of deformity.

MACHINE USE FOR MASSAGE

1. Manipulator
2. Neurotripsor [hand held device] for local area.
3. Suction wave massage
4. Stationary device [vibrating belt]

5. Intermittent depression system.
6. Massage roller peg
7. Flotrons
8. Lymph mat
9. External winter pulsation
10. Shower massage

11

TRACTION

DEFINITION

It is basically, a technique in which distractive force is applied on the body or body parts. An effort is applied to separate joint especially for the purpose to increase joint range of motion. Joint range of motion helps to mobility of the joint & relief from arthopathy. It is a system of force applied to body along its length. (Fig. 11.1).

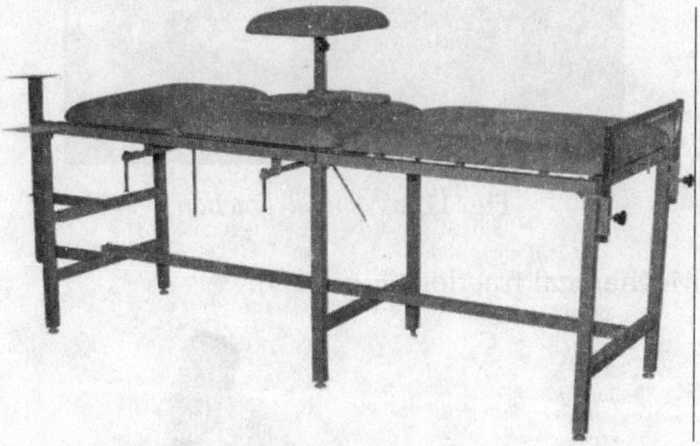

Fig. 11.1: *Traction Table*

Types of Traction

Three types of traction on the basis of structural changes:

Stage 1st – Mild force without separation of joint

Stage2nd – Actual separation of the joint

Stage 3rd – Involved soft tissue broken off & distractive forces applied.

Type of traction on the basis of duration

Continuous traction: this type of traction is used for temporary immobilization of part, used low force for hours to days.

Sustained traction: in this traction force is slight greater than that used in continues traction. It is for 20-60 minutes.

Intermittent traction: in this traction technique greater force used for short period of time, this force increased and decreased during treatment cycle.

Type of traction on the basis of force application

- Manual traction (Fig. 11.2).

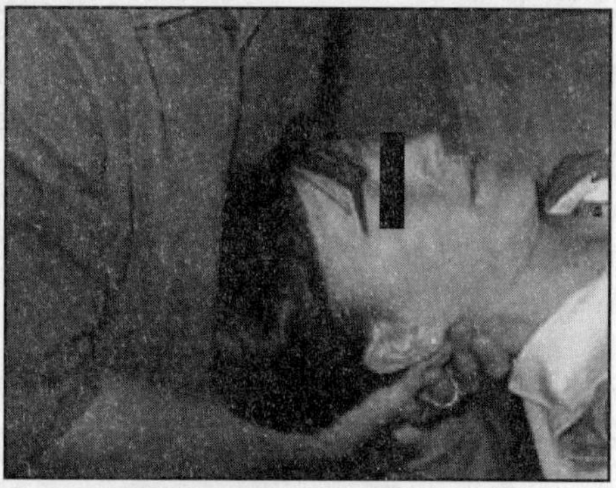

Fig. 11.2: *Manual Traction*

- Mechanical traction (Fig. 11.3).

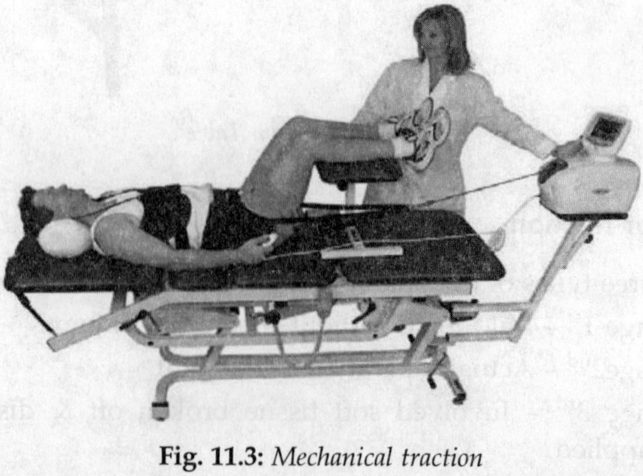

Fig. 11.3: *Mechanical traction*

- Positional Traction (Fig. 11.4)

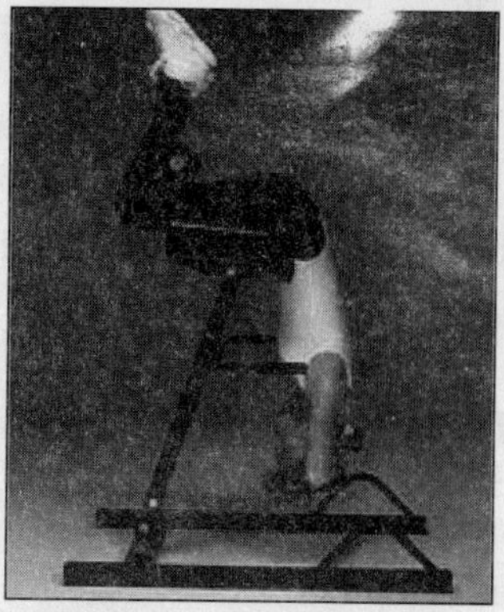

Fig. 11.4: *Positional Traction*

PRINCIPLE OF APPLIED FORCE

- Force of sufficient magnitude & distraction should be applied.
- Direction of traction force should be in the line with the longitudinal axis of joint to be treated.
- Position of patient should be sitting, lying or standing.
- A counter traction i.e. an equal and opposite force to that of traction force must be applied, so that the efficient distraction at the joint surface occurs.

EFFECTS

- Distraction
- Suction effect
- Ligament lengthening
- Relief in muscle spasm
- Relief from pain
- Facilitation of nerve injury
- Enlargement of intervertebral space
- Space increase between intervertebral discs
- Stretching of joint capsule

INDICATIONS

- Arthritis
- Soft tissue contracture
- Joint space narrowing
- Fracture where bony tissues are malaligned
- Spinal disorder

CONTRAINDICATIONS

- Old persons
- Tuberculosis of spine
- Osteoporosis
- Tumor
- Osteomyelitis
- Pregnancy
- Respiratory problem
- Old & weak patient
- Rheumatoid arthritis
- Severe anxiety
- Myelopathy (Destruction of muscle fibres)
- Spinal stenosis (Fusion of vertebrae)
- Spine instability (Spondylolisthesis)

12

SUSPENSION

Suspension therapy is given by basically a frame unit including ropes, pulleys and sling. This frame is also known as Guthrie Smith frame. (Fig. 12.1).

Suspension is that in which parts of body are supported in slings & elevated by use of variable-length-ropes which are fixed to a point (hook) above the body. It permits free movement without resistance. It frees the body from the friction of material, upon which body components may be resting.

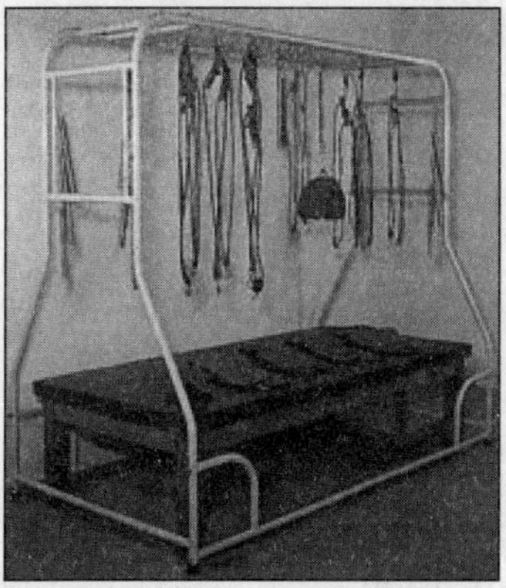

Fig. 12.1: *Suspension apparatus (Guthrie Smith Frame)*

PARTS OF SUSPENSION

The Fixed Point

It is use to suspend the overhead mesh from ceiling joints at a height which will allow about 1.5 m clearance between mesh and plinth top.

Storage

Storage of slings and ropes can be on a wall frame of suitable hooks with large and small curves.

The Supporting Ropes

Ropes should be of 3-ply hemp as they are non-slippery. Ropes can be arranged in three ways:

1. Single rope—It has a ring, fixed at one end by which it is hung up. The other end of rope passes through one end of a wooden cleat and is then knotted with a half hitch. The cleat is for altering the length of rope.
2. Pulley rope—It has a dog clip attached to one end
3. Double rope.

Slings

They are of 4 types:

1. Single slings
2. Double slings
3. Three ring slings
4. Head slings

Clips

Karabiner hooks of 70 mm or 100 mm provide a convenient alternative means of clipping two pieces of equipment together.

TYPES OF SUSPESION

1. Vertical Suspension
2. Axial Suspension
3. Pendular Suspension

Vertical Suspension

- In vertical suspension, the rope is fixed vertically, hangs above the centre of gravity of suspended part.
- Vertical suspension is used for support and to limit the movement of part to a small range pendulum movement

on each side of central resting point.

- In other words, the support is partly lost and the movement is limited by length of ropes. It is used primarily to support, e.g. the abducted upper limb when the elbow is to be moved is supported from above the centre of gravity of the arm and axial fixation is used over the elbow for forearm movement.

Axial Suspension

- When all ropes are supporting a part with 'S 'hook and attached to a fixed point, immediately above the centre of joint which is to be moved.
- When such fixation is set up, the movement of the limb will be on a flat plane level with the floor. In this way pure angular movements are obtained.
- The whole fix point may move away from muscles which require resistance for requirement of some resistance to the muscle work.

Pendular Suspension

It is a type of suspension in which the axis of axial suspension is changed to apply resistance to a moving limb. The axis is shifted away from the axial fixation of the hip joint (e.g.- Patient lies in side lying the axis of the suspension is shifted posterior to the hip joint to strengthen the flexors of the hip joint).

USE OF SUSPENSIONS

A. Suspension for the Lower Extremity

1. *The Hip joint*

Abduction and Adduction: Type of suspension is axial - In axial suspension the patient is supine lying, the unaffected extremity is abducted at hip joint and flexed at knee joint, the foot is placed on stool. The placement of 'S' hook, ropes and sling are fixed immediately over the hip joint on which two ropes are suspended. (Fig. 12.2).

The length of ropes is altered by the movement of the cleat until the limb is lifted horizontal. The patient is then allowed to move the hip joint in abduction and adduction.

Type of suspension is vertical—In vertical suspension, the patient is in supine lying, the unaffected limb is abducted at hip and flexed at knee joint, the foot is placed on the stool. For vertical suspension the 'S' hook is placed immediately over the center of gravity of the thigh and is attached with the rope than the sling of the knee joint. As vertical fixation is often combined with axial fixation, therefore one S is also placed just above the hip joint and is attached with rope. The three ring sling supports the foot and ankle and its center ring is attached with rope. The length of rope is altered by the movement of cleat until the limb comes in horizontal line than patient is allowed to move the joint in abduction and adduction.

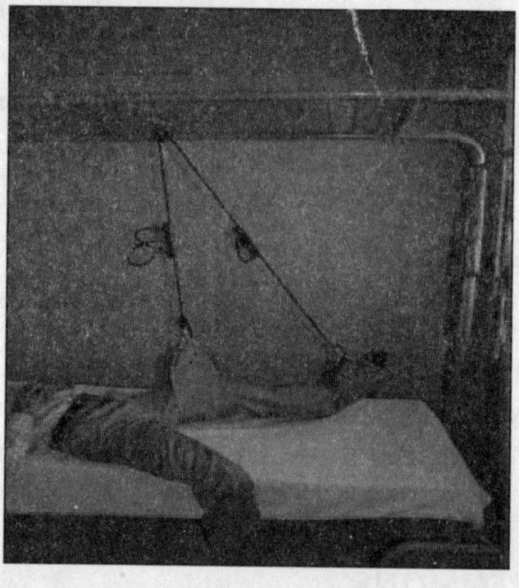

Fig. 12.2: *Hip joint abduction and adduction*

Flexion and Extension

- ***Type of suspension is axial***—The patient is in side lying position, the lower leg or unaffected leg is flexed at hip and knee joint. For axial suspension the 'S' hook is fixed immediately over the hip joint on which two ropes are suspended. The two slings at knee and ankle joint are attached with the D rings and then dog clip and ropes. The length of rope is altered by the movement of cleat until the limb comes in horizontal line than patient is allowed to move the joint in flexion and extension. (Fig.

12.3a- 12.3b).

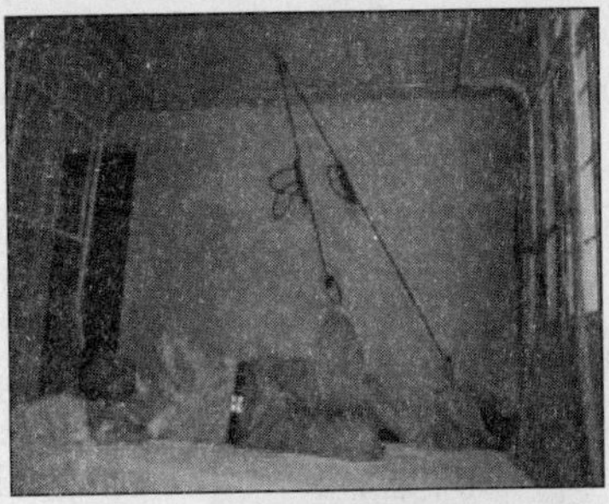

Fig. 12.3a: *Hip joint flexion*

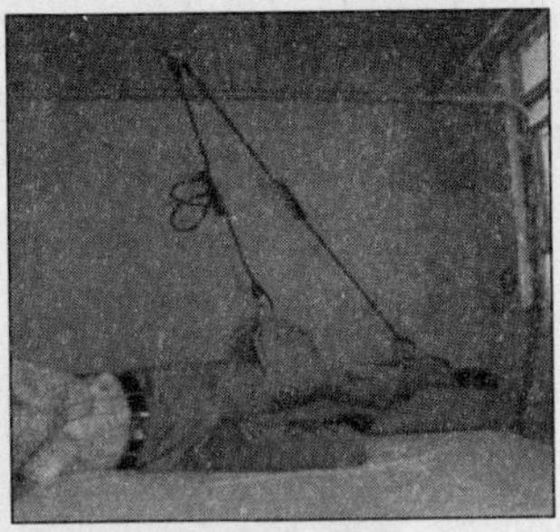

Fig. 12.3b: *Hip joint extension*

Type of suspension is vertical—The patient is in side lying position, the lower leg or unaffected leg is flexed at hip and knee joint. For vertical suspension the 'S' hook is placed immediately over the center of gravity of the thigh and is attached with the rope than the sling of the knee joint. As vertical fixation is often combined with axial fixation, therefore one S is also placed just above the hip joint and is attached with rope. The three ring sling supports the foot and ankle and its center ring is attached with rope. The length of rope is altered by the movement of cleat until the limb comes in horizontal line than patient is allowed to move the joint in flexion and extension.

2. ***The Knee Joint***

Flexion and Extension: *Type of suspension is axial*—The patient is in side lying position (Fig. 12.4). Axis on the knee joint.

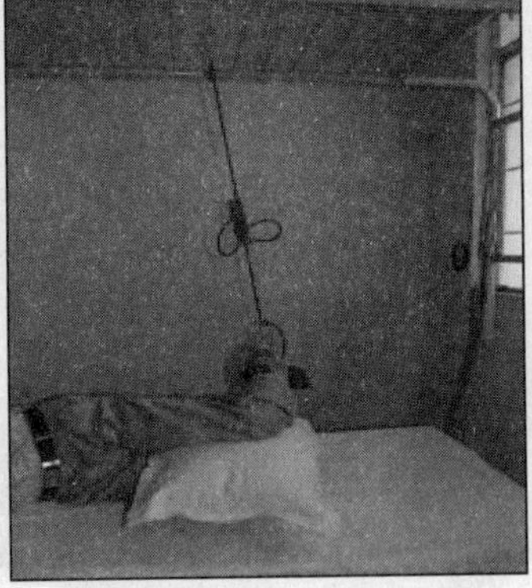

Fig. 12.4 : *The knee joint flexion and extension*

B. Suspension For The Upper Extremity

1. The Shoulder Joint

Abduction and Adduction: Type of suspension is axial—The patient is in supine lying position. (Fig. 12.5)

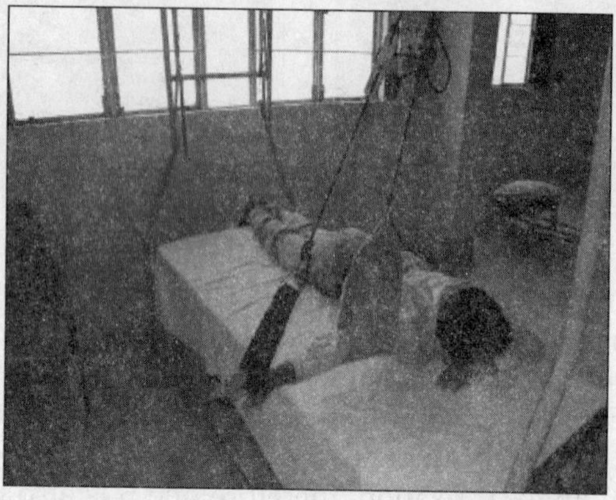

Fig. 12.5: *The Shoulder joint abduction and adduction*

Flexion and Extension: Type of suspension is axial - The patient is in side lying position. (Fig. 12.6)

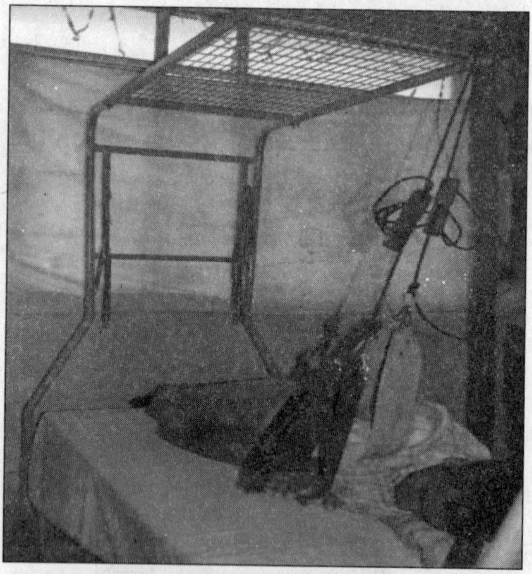

Fig. 12.6: *The Shoulder joint flexion and extension*

2. ***The Elbow Joint***

Flexion and Extension: Type of suspension is axial - The patient is in sitting position. (Fig. 12.7)

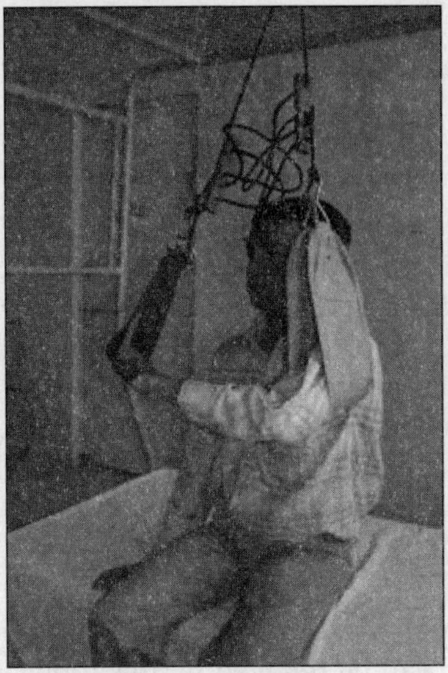

Fig. 12.7: *The Elbow joint flexion and extension*

13

RELAXATION

Relaxation is a condition of muscle in which relaxed muscles have relatively decreased tension or tone and are at rest. Various conditions require appropriate relaxation technique such as state of fatigue, neuromuscular conditions, hypertension, stress, sleep disturbances, pre and post operative conditions, spasticity, Bell's palsy, burns etc.

MUSCLE TENSION AND MUSCLE TONE

The tension of muscles can be affected by conscious effort and thought and can be relieved by the application of conscious thought or muscular effort on the affected part of the patient. The difference between tension and relaxation may be observed for example, in the difference in posture of an athlete at then beginning of a sprint start and that at the end of the race when the line has been crossed or in the learner driver who sits tenses and hunched over the steering wheel as opposed to the relaxation of the accustomed and experienced driver. Muscle tone, which represents a state of preparedness in resting muscles, is now thought to be maintained through the activity of muscle spindle circuit. The efferent fibres of this small fiber nervous reflex pathway transmit impulses which produce a sustained contraction of the small intrafusal muscle fibres of muscle spindles, while the large extrafusal fibres concerned with voluntary movement remain relaxed.

VOLUNTARY MOVEMENT

Specific muscle contracts and then initiate or controls the movement to do the work and finally at the completion of movement they come to rest or relaxed state. Contraction in any one group of muscles is accompanied by a reciprocal relaxation of antagonistic group to allow movement to take place smoothly. It has importance in designing the methods to obtain relaxation of a particular group of muscle.

MENTAL ATTITUDE

Fear, anger and excitement give rise to increase in muscular tension which results in the rapid and forceful action. The therapist reassures the patient and gain his confidence via cooperation and provide atmosphere for physical and mental rest, which helps the patient to acquire the art of voluntary relaxation. This voluntary relaxation helps the patient to economies the nervous energy.

PATHOLOGICAL TENSION IN MUSCLE

A persistent increase in muscular tension or tone is a feature of many pathological conditions which affects the nervous system. Lesions of higher motor centers results in abnormal state of muscular tension which may vary from hypertonicity to spasticity or rigidity. A temporary reduction in this tension in the affected area can be achieved by promoting relaxation and it is useful in re-education of any functional activity which remains to take place.

TECHNIQUE OF RELAXATION

1. Local Relaxation

- Massage
- Passive movement
- Hold relax
- Contract relax

2. General Relaxation

- By support
- By comfort

- By restful atmosphere
- By Contrast method
- By Breathing consciously.

OTHER RELAXATION TECHNIQUE

Local Relaxation

Methods of obtaining local relaxation depends to some extent on the cause and distribution of the tension.

Massage

Relaxation of a specific area is obtained by the application of the general principles of massage already described for the whole body or to that area. A general attitude of rest will however assist the process e.g. limbs are the abducted and flexed when the patient lies or reclines in a chair, this is followed by sitting upright.

Passive Movement

More beneficial than stretching the muscle when it is performed on particular muscle or group of muscle. Rhythmical passive movement of the limbs and head may assist the degree of general relaxation in some cases these movements are generally given as a sequel to massage. Group movements of joints, e.g. flexion and extension of hip, knee and ankle are preferable, but a very high standard of performance on the part of the physiotherapist is required to obtain results, the rhythm of small pendular movements pleases some patients. The ability to promote a state of relaxation depends very largely on the individual physiotherapist and the particular patient with whom she is dealing, and details of successful methods employed vary widely ideal conditions are rarely obtainable and, indeed are hardly desirable for many patient must eventually learn to relax where and when the opportunity present itself e.g. in the train or an mountain top after a strenuous climb.

Hold Relax

This technique consists of offering resistance to a muscle / muscles group which is in tension. The patient is commanded to hold the limb in position while the therapist applies equal resistance against the patient's contraction, this produces isometric contraction of the tense muscle. No movement should occur, when the therapist feels that the patient has reached the limits of his potential contraction. He should grasp the limb firmly but comfortably and at the same time asks the patient to relax to let go and allow some time to elapse which is at least as long as or perhaps longer than the time taken to build up the maximum contraction .This technique is of special use when a patient has no movement because of pain - spasm.

Contract Relax

This technique may be used when a patient has a small range of motion and is prevented from moving further by the spasm of muscle.

The patient is asked to move the joint in pain free range. This range may also be achieved by passive movement, therapist grasp, the limb and patient is then asked to make a small strongly isotonic resisted contraction back to the original position. At the end of movement the part is grasped firmly but comfortably and the patient is told to relax.

GENERAL RELAXATION

By Support

Various forms and modifications of the lying position are used to achieve full support of the body, the relative suitability of each one varying according to the condition of the patient and to individual preference.

Supine Lying

Lying comfortably on weight/couch with full support to each part of the body. A head pillow is required which is sufficiently soft to prevent the head from rolling to either side, and to be well moulded to support the neck posteriorly. A small pillow under the knees relives tension on the hamstrings and the iliofemoral ligament and consequently allows the pelvis to roll backwards so that the lumber spine is straightened and supported. The feet are held in the mid position by a sand bag or similar device and each arm slightly abducted at the shoulder and flexed at the elbow, rests on a pillow.

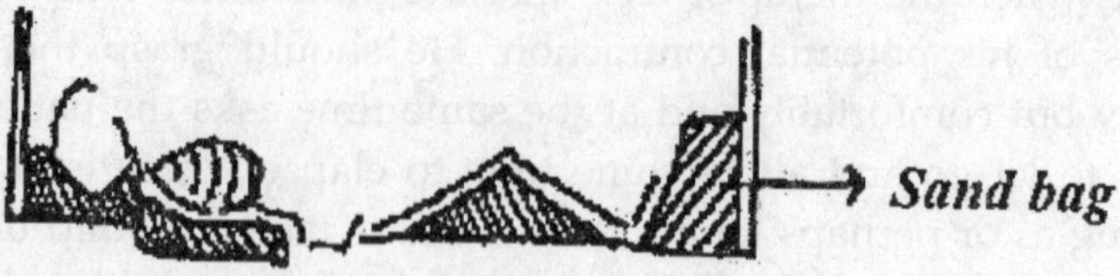

Fig. 13.1: *Supine lying*

Half Lying

This is similar to the previous position but breathing is easier as there is less weight on the back and abdominal pressure. An armchair makes quite a good substitute for plinth or bed, the thighs are fully supported and the feet rest on the floor, or a footstool.

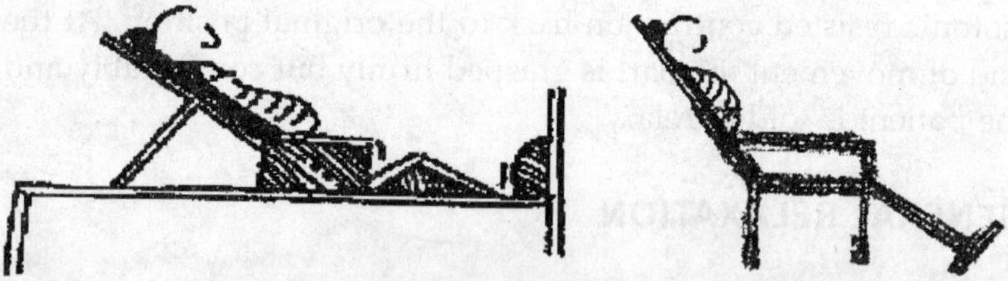

Fig. 13.2: *Half lying*

Prone Lying

The head is turned to one side and may rest on a small pillow, if more comfortable, a firm pillow under the hips and the lower abdomen prevents hollowing of the back, and for women it should extend higher to avoid too much pressure on the back, the lower leg is elevated so that the knees are slightly bent and the toes relaxed. A degree of medial rotation at the hips, causing the heel to fall apart still further induces relaxation of the legs. Many find this position comfortable and use it for sleeping; others dislike it because of the rotated position of the head. (Fig. 13.3)

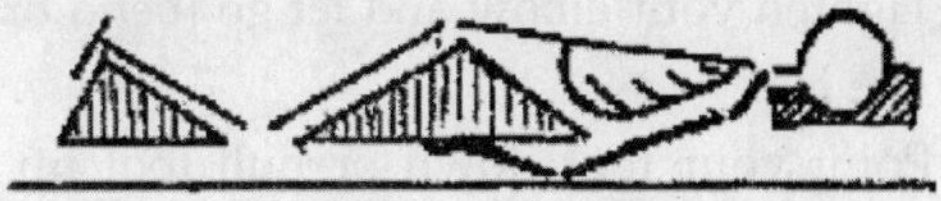

Fig. 13.3: *Prone lying*

The measure of relaxation obtained is governed by the efficiency with which the shoulder and pelvic girdles is stabilized. The arm and leg which is uppermost may be rested on the supporting surface instead of a pillow but some of the weight then falls on the trunk ands this impedes respiration. The head pillow supports the neck and head in alignment with the body, and must not be too high. Suitable positioning plays important role in promoting relaxation.

By Comfort

In comfort well balance meal, rhythmical physical activity brisk walk in the open air and individual positioning are required. Comfort also include freedom to breathe deeply, warmth and removal of constrictive cloths (E.g.- Tight belt, buttons etc).

By Restful Atmosphere

The treatment – room should be as quiet as possible, a many people for whom training in relaxation is prescribed are highly susceptible to the disturbing influence of noise.

By Contrast Method

This includes often be taught by demonstrating the contrast between maximal contraction and the degree of relaxation which follows it, the patient being told to contract any group of series of muscles as strongly as possible and then to let go and continue to let go.

The sequence of commands is as follows (alternative or explanatory commands are in brackets)-

1. For the arm-
    - Make a fist and let go.
    - Tighten your wrist and let go (pull your hands back or forwards).

- Tighten your elbow and let go (bend or straighten).

2. For the leg-
   - Point your foot down or pull foot up and let go,(the patient chooses whichever is least likely to give him cramp).
   - Tighten your knee and let go, (straighten your knees).
   - Tighten your hips and let go, (Tightens the buttock).
3. For the trunk and head-
   - Press your head against your support and let go.
   - Press your shoulders against your support and let go.

Deep breathing may be practiced with relaxation of any part of the body, it is more usual to breathe in while tensing the muscles and to breathe out on letting go.

By Breathing Consciously

Under conditions of quiet and comfort the patient's mind may remain active and turn to mundane problems and anxieties with associated physical tension, In case it may help to concentrate on his rhythm of breathing, which must be deep with a slight pause at the end of expiration. Expiration is a phase of relaxation and should be accompanied by a feeling of letting go in the whole body.

OTHER RELAXATION TECHNIQUES

- Yoga and meditation
- Recreational therapy
- Music therapy
- Pet therapy
- Pool therapy
- Social therapy
- Biofeedback
- Jacobson's progressive relaxation technique

■

14

ACTIVITIES OF DAILY LIVING

CONCEPT OF ADL & I-ADL

Daily activities can be separated in to two areas namely basic activities of daily living and instrumental activities of daily living. ADL requires basic skills whereas Instrumental ADL (I-ADL) requires more advanced problem solving skills, social skills and more complex environmental interactions.

CLASSIFICATION

Basic ADL.

- **Mobility:** Bed & wheelchair mobility, transfers and ambulation.
- **Self care:** Dressing, self feeding, toileting grooming, bathing etc.
- **Communication**: Writing, typing, telephone, etc.
- **Environmental hardware:** Keys, faucets, switches windows etc.

Instrumental ADL.

- Home management: Shopping, meal preparation,laundry child care etc.
- Community living skills: Driving, public transport, etc
- Health management: Handling medicines, knowing health risks etc.

- Safety management: fire safety awareness, safety symbols, making emergency calls etc.
- Environmental hardware: vacuum cleaner, refrigerator, oven

EVALUATION

- Evaluation of client.
- Evaluation of the environment of client.

Therapist assesses not only the client but also his/ her surroundings. Home visits, interview of client and family/ neighbours, observation of client while performing various tasks, discussions with other rehabilitation team members etc. are commonly used by therapist for ADL assessment. There are various standard instruments for assessing physical and/ or multidimensional functions e.g. Barthel index, Katz index of ADL, Functional independence measure (FIM), Sickness impact profile (SIP) etc.

INTERVENTIONS

Approaches

1. Remedial
2. Adaptive
3. Educational

Intervention Instruments

Assistive devices e.g. long handled comb, dressing stick (Fig. 14.1), scooped disc, cuffed spoon (14.2), angulated spoon (Fig. 14.3) etc.

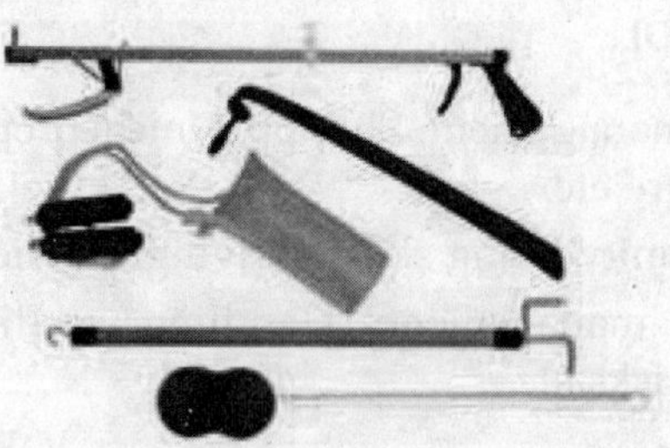

Fig.: *Dressing stick*

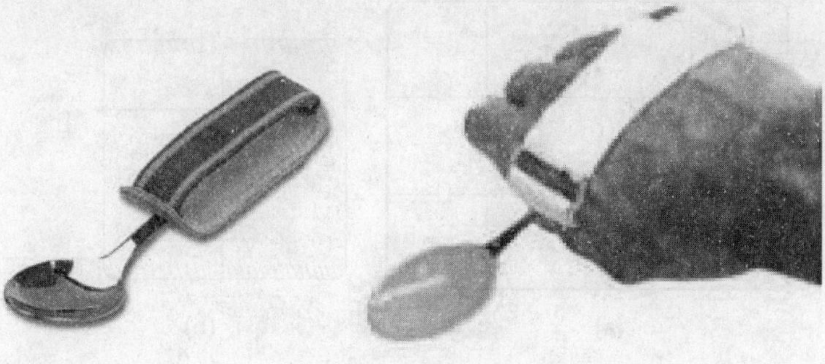

Fig. 14.2: *Cuffed spoon*

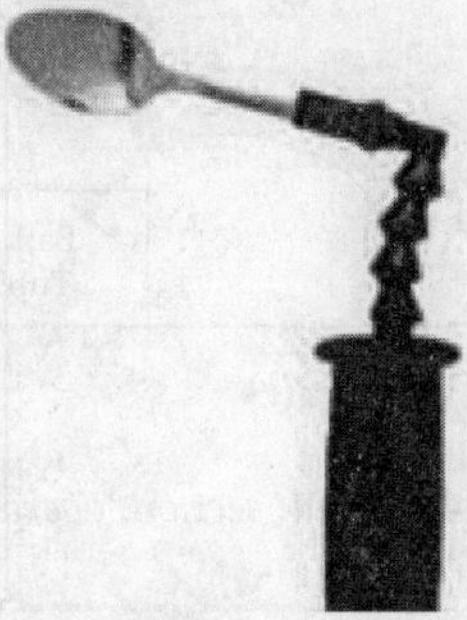

Fig. 14.3: *Angulated spoon*

1. Teaching ADL e.g. backward/forward chaining methods of teaching.
2. Specific ADL techniques for daily activities e.g. dressing, grooming, eating etc.
3. Mat, bed, wheel chair and upright (cane, crutches, orthoses etc.) activities.

ADL room (Fig 14.4) is specially designed for training purposes, imparting functional independence to needy clients. An ideal ADL room consist of various segments e.g. feeding section, bathing section, dressing section, toilet section etc.

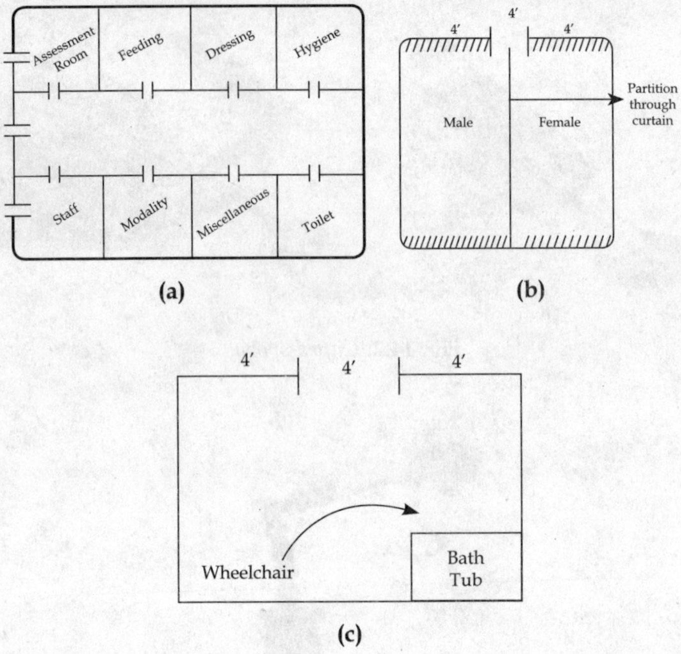

Fig. 14.4: *ADL section: overview*

SCOPE OF ADLs

A person with physical and mental disability needs many changes that lead to independence in ADLs. A therapist needs to do:

- Careful assessment
- Goal setting
- Planning

Training is important for goal setting for self sufficiency in ADLs as it causes—

- Dependency
- Frustration
- Hyperirritability

Training is important in acute case also. It is important in disability condition like –

- Multiple sclerosis
- Hemeplegia
- Parkinson disease

PROFORMA FOR ADLS

Grading should be done while completion of ADL Performa.

(a) Independent grading

Grade 4 – Normal performance.

Grade 3 – Alternative performance but dependent on special apparatus or environmental factors.

(b) Depending grading

Grade 2 - Needed complete supervision

Grade 1 - Needed complete assistance

Grade x - Not presenting

Grade NA - Not available

ASSESSMENT PROFORMA FOR ADLs

a. Individual Data

Name

Age / sex

Address

Occupation

Dominance

OPD number

Diagnosis

Examiner

b. Individual's ADLs data

Activity	Grade	Remark
(A) Locomotors activity		
Bed mobility		
Sit on the bed		
Transfer from bed to wheelchair		
Transfer from wheelchair to bed		

Transfer from wheelchair to toilet
Transfer from toilet to wheelchair
Transfer from wheelchair to car
Wheelchair by himself
Wheelchair use on ramp
Pick up the objects floor
Close or open the door
Walk backward
Walk sideways
Stair climbing
Walk with holding objects
Riding and getting from bus

(B) ***Eating activity***

Eat himself
Drink water through glass
Drink water through cup
Drink water through bottle
Drink water through straw
Eat with spoon
Eat with fork
Cut through knife
Cut through sickle

(C) ***Hygiene activity***

Brushing
Use of handkerchief
Hand wash
Face wash
Hair combing
Care for nails
Make up
Shampooing
Shaving
Use of perfume and deodorant

Bathing
Use of hair oil
Care of menstrual period

(D) Dressing activity

Put on or Put off cardigan and sweater
Put on or Put off shirt and pant
Put on or Put off salwar suit
Put on or Put off coat
Put on or Put off trouser
Put on or Put off socks
Put on or Put off tie
Put on or Put off brassier
Put on or Put off undergarments / lingerie
Lock unlock well crow
Tie laces
Use of accessories

(E) Environmental Hardware

Use of switches of fan and others
Operate toilet flux
Open and close drawer
Operate locks
Playing cards
Use of telephone
Use of key board
Use of musical instrument
Prepare chapatti
Use of grinder
Use of iron
Washing cloths

(F) Communication activity

Through writing
Through telephone
Through SMS

Through internet
Through E – mail
Through fax
Through letter sending
Through body language
Through speech

(G) Play activity

15

ASSISTIVE DEVICES AND GAIT PATTERNS

Before continuing with the progression of gait training activities outside the parallel bars, following assistive devices may be used-

1. Walker
2. Canes
3. Crutches

WALKER

Walkers are used to improve balance and relieve weight bearing either fully or partially on a lower extremity. It helps in -

- Wide B.O.S.
- Improve anterior and lateral stability
- Allow the upper extremity to transfer body weight to the floor

These are made up of aluminium pipe with molded vinyl handgrips and rubber tips. They are adjusted according to children, adult size with respect to height. Several modifications available in standard design are as follows:-

1. A folding mechanism in walker
2. Handgrips
3. Platform attachment
4. Reciprocal walker
5. Wheel attachment
6. Stair climbing walkers

7. Baskets
8. Seating surface
9. Glides

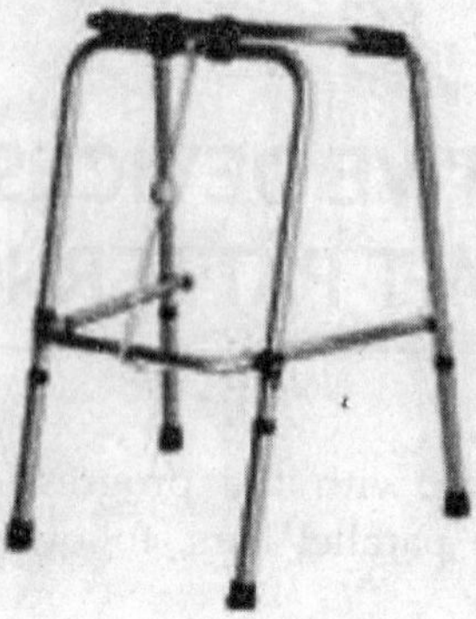

Fig. 15.1: *Walker*

Advantages of Walker

- Walkers provide four points of floor contact with a wide BOS.
- They provide a high level of stability
- They provide sense of security against fearful ambulation
- They are relatively lightweight & easily adjusted

Disadvantages of Walker

- Walker tends to be cumbersome
- Awkward in confined areas
- Difficult to maneuver through doorways & into cars
- They eliminate normal arm swing
- It can't be used safely on stairs

Measurement for Walkers

- Walker should come to the level of greater trochanter.
- It should allow 20 to 30 degrees of elbow flexion.
- To measure the walker height, the center of a broad based walker is placed approximately 6 inches from

lateral border of toes. The top of walker should come at the level of greater trochanter & elbow should be flexed to 20 to 30 degrees. Elbow flexion allows the arm to shorten or to lengthen during different phase of gait and it provides a shock absorption mechanism.

Gait Patterns : Walker

There are three types of gait patterns used with walkers as follows:-

1. Full weight bearing gait
2. Partial weight bearing gait
3. Non weight bearing gait

Full Weight Bearing Gait

- The walker is picked up and moved forward about an arm's length.
- First lower extremity is moved forward.
- Second lower extremity is moved forward past the first.

Partial Weight Bearing Gait

- The walker is picked up and moved forward about an arm's length.
- The involved lower extremity is moved forward and body weight is transferred partially onto this limb and partially through the upper extremities to the walker.
- The uninvolved lower extremity is moved forward past the involved limb.
- The cycle is repeated.

Non-weight Bearing Gait

- The walker is picked up and moved forward about an arm's length.
- Weight is transferred through upper extremities to the walker. The involved limb is held anterior to the patient's body but does not make contact with the floor.
- The uninvolved limb is moved forward.

- The cycle is repeated.

CANES

These are constructed of lightweight aluminium. The function of a cane is to widen the Base of support and to improve balance.

1. Standard Cane

These are constructed of aluminium, wood, plastic. They have a half circle (crook) handle. The distal rubber tip is at least 1 inch in diameter.

Advantages

This cane is inexpensive and fits easily on stairs or other surfaces where space is limited.

Disadvantage

The standard cane is not adjustable and must be cut to fit the patient. Its point of support is anterior to the hand not directly beneath it.

2. Standard Adjustable Aluminium Cane

It is made of aluminium tubing and has a half circle handle with a molded plastic covering.

Measurement

The height to be adjusted by placing the locking pin mechanism into the proper notch and within the range of 27 to 38.5 inches (68 to 98 cm). The distal rubber tip is at least 1 inch in diameter.

Advantage

- This cane is quickly adjustable, facilitating ease of determining appropriate height.
- It is particularly useful for measurement prior to altering the length of a standard cane.
- It is lightweight and fits easily on stairs.

Disadvantage

- The point of support is anterior to the hand, not directly beneath it.
- This cane is more costly than a standard cane.

3. Adjustable Aluminium Offset Cane

The shaft of this cane is offset anteriorly creating a straight or offset handle. It is made up of aluminium tubing with a plastic or rubber molded grip shaped handle.

Measurement

- The height to be adjusted from 27 to 38.5 inches (68 to 98 cm) by a pin or notch mechanism.
- The diameter of distal rubber tip is at least 1 inch.

Advantages

- The design of this cane allows pressure to be borne over the center of cane for greater stability.
- This cane also is quickly adjusted, lightweight and fits easily on stairs.

Disadvantages

- This cane is costlier than standard or adjustable aluminium cane.

4. Quadruped Cane

This constructed of aluminium and aluminium tubing. Both large based quad canes and small-based quad canes are commercially available. They provide a broad base with 4 points of floor contact. Each point is covered with rubber tip. Its height is adjusted from 28 to 38 inches (71 to 91 cm).

Advantages

- This cane provides a broad based support.
- Bases are available in several different sizes.
- This cane is also easily adjustable.

Disadvantages

- The patient's hand pressure may not be centered over the cane and may result instability.

- As a result of broad BOS, some quad canes may not be practical for use of stairs.

They warrant use of a slower gait pattern. If a faster forward progression is used, the cane often "rocks" from rear legs to front legs, which decreases effectiveness of the cane.

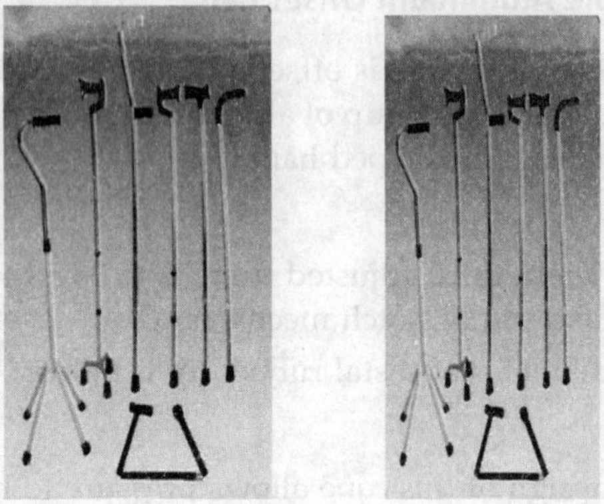

Fig. 15.2: *Walking sticks* *Quadruped, tripods*

Advantages

- Walk canes provide very broad based support and are more stable than a quad cane.
- These canes also fold flat for travel or storage.

Disadvantages

- Specific design of a walk cane or hand grip placement may not pressure to be centered over the cane.
- Walk canes cannot be used on most stairs.
- They require use of a slow forward progression and are generally costlier than quad canes.

Hand Grips

The type of handgrip should be judge and selected primarily on the basis of patient comfort and on the grips ability to provide adequate surface area to allow effective transfer of weight from upper extremity to floor. The more common types of handgrips are-

1. The crook handle

2. The straight / offset handle
3. The shovel handle
4. The pistol handle

Types of Handle Grips

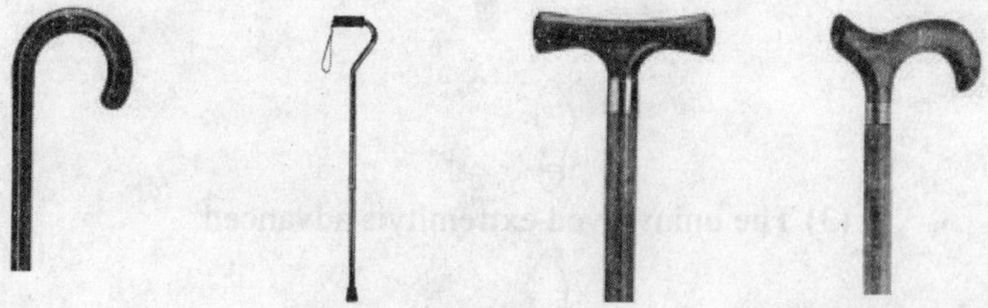

1 2 3 4

Measurement

Cane height, is measured from greater trochanter of femur to the floor approximately 6 inches Lateral to lateral boarder of the toes and 2 inches anterior. (Fig. 15.3)

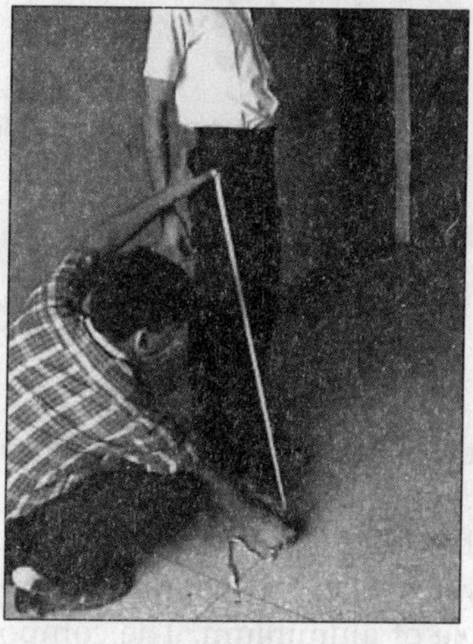

Fig. 15.3: *Measurement of cane*

Gait Patterns : Cane

For ambulation on level surfaces, the cane should be held in the upper extremity opposite to the affected limb. The cane and the affected limb both are advanced simultaneously. The cane should be held close to the body and should not be placed ahead of the toe of the affected limb.

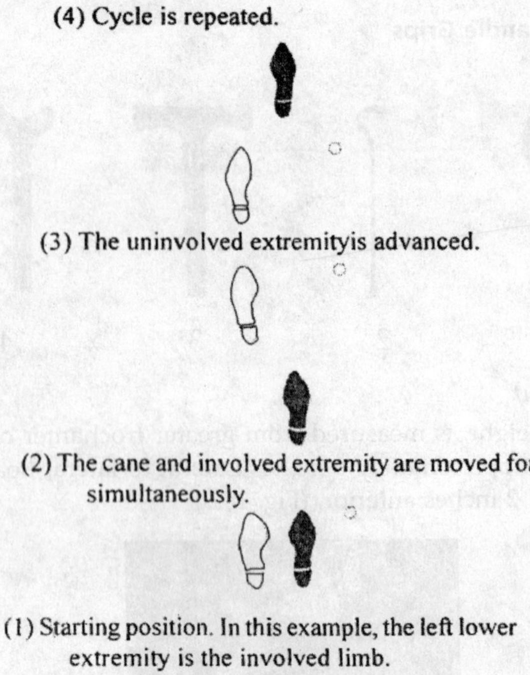

Fig. 15.4: *Gait Pattern Using Cane*

CRUTCHES

Crutches are commonly used to relieve weight either partially or fully on lower extremities. Two type of crutches i.e. axillary crutches (Fig 15.5) and elbow crutches or forearm crutches. Axillary crutches are commonly made up of wood but it also available of aluminium. The components of standard axillary crutches are axillary bar, hand piece, double upright joined distally by a single leg and rubber suction tip.

Axillary crutches are difficult to use in crowded areas as they require larger base of support. (Fig. 15.5) Neuropraxia in axilla is the common complication of improper use of axillary crutches.

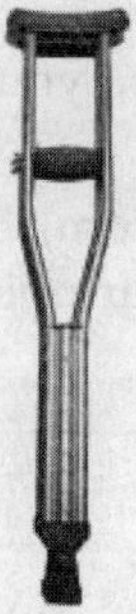

Fig. 15.5: *Axillary crutch*

Measurement of Axillary Crutches

In standing position measurement is taken from 2 inches below the axilla to the point on floor 2 inches lateral and 6 inches anterior to the toes while in supine from axillary fold to a point on plinth 6-8 inches lateral to the heel. (Fig. 15.6)

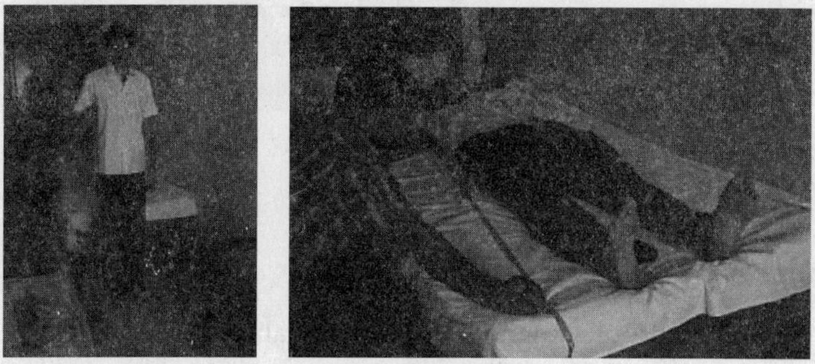

(a) (b)

Fig. 15.6: *Measurement of axillary crutch in standing position (a) and supine lying (b) position*

Even if you've already been fitted with crutches, make sure your crutch pads and handgrips are set at the proper distance (fig.15.6), as follows:

- Crutch pad distance from armpits. The crutch pads (tops of crutches) should be 1.5″ to 2″ (about two finger widths) below the armpits, with the shoulders relaxed.

- Handgrip. Place it so your elbow is flexed about 20 to 30 degrees—enough so you can fully extend your elbow when you take a step.

Crutch length (top to bottom). The total crutch length should equal the distance from your armpit to about 6" in front of shoe.

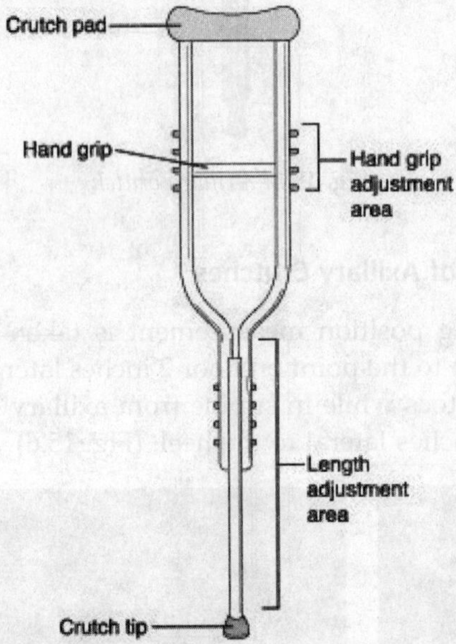

Fig. 15.7: *Crutch length*

Important Rules for Safety and Comfort

- Don't look down. Look straight ahead as you normally do when you walk.
- Don't use crutches if you feel dizzy or drowsy.
- Don't walk on slippery surfaces. Avoid snowy, icy, or rainy conditions.
- Don't put any weight on your foot if your doctor has so advised.
- Do make sure your crutches have rubber tips.
- Do wear well-fitting, low-heel shoes (or shoe).
- Do position the crutch handgrips correctly (see "Sizing Your Crutches")

- Do keep the crutch pads 11/2" to 2" below your armpits.
- Do call your foot and ankle surgeon if you have any questions or difficulties.

Gait Pattern

An appropriate gait pattern is determined by the amount of weight bearing permitted and the severity of the patient's condition.

Commonly used gait patterns include swing to, swing through, four point, three point, and two point.

Two Point Gait

Used to describe a pattern in which a patient used two crutches or canes. The patient ambulates moving the left crutch forward while simultaneously advancing the right lower extremity and vice - versa. Each step is "one point" and a complete cycle is two points. (Fig. 15.8)

Three Point Gait

This pattern can be seen with a walker, crutches, or cans. It involves one injured lower extremity that may have decreased weight bearing. The assistive device is advanced followed by the injured lower extremity and then the uninjured lower extremity. The assistive device and each lower extremity are considered separate points. (Fig. 15.8)

Four Point Gait

This pattern is very similar to the two point pattern. The primary difference is that in this pattern patient does not move the lower extremities simultaneously, but waits and advances the opposite leg once the crutch/cane has been advanced. The gait pattern may be prescribed when a patient exhibits impaired coordination, balance, and significant strength deficits. Each advancement of the crutch or cane as well as the bilateral lower extremities indicates a single point, thus allowing for four-point gait pattern. (Fig. 15.8)

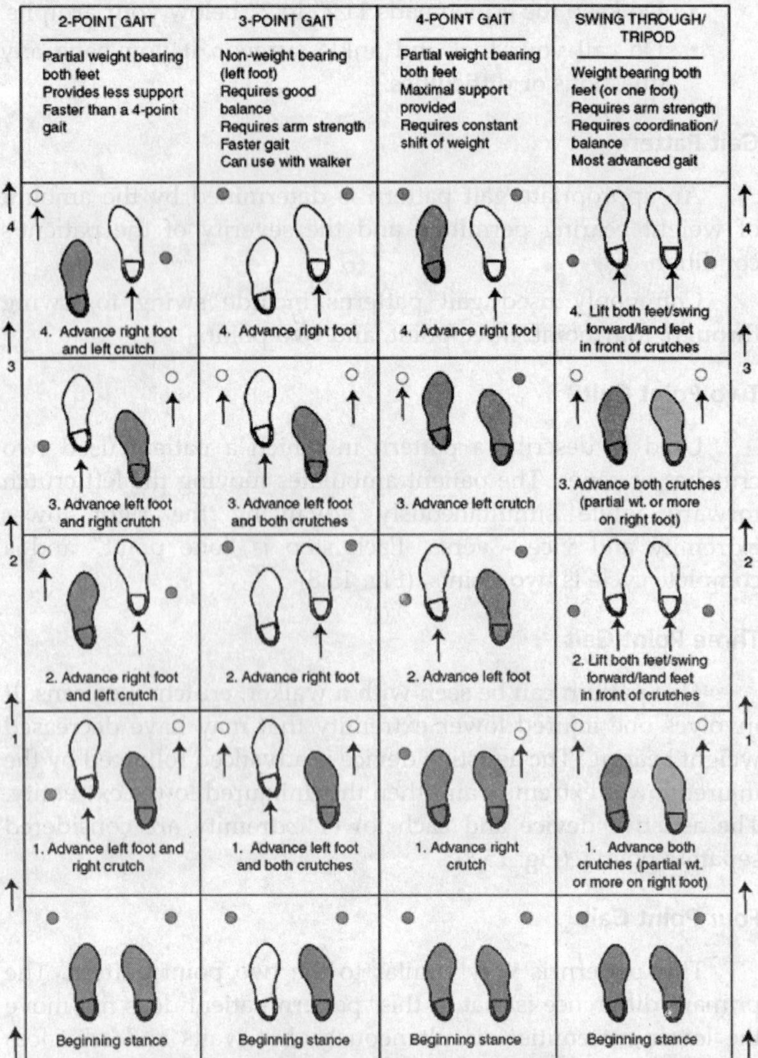

Fig. 15.8: *Gait pattern*

The gait pattern may be prescribed when a patient exhibits impaired coordination, balance, and significant strength deficits. Each advancement of the crutch or cane as well as the bilateral lower extremities indicates a single point, thus allowing for four-point gait pattern.

Swing to Gait

A style of gait where a patient uses crutches or a walker and advances the lower extremities simultaneously only to the point of the assistive device.

Swing through Gait

This patient performs the same sequence as a swing to gait pattern, however advances the lower extremities beyond the point of the assistive device.

■

16

ACTIVE AND PASSIVE MOVEMENT

MOVEMENT

1. Active Movement

A. *Voluntary movement.*

a. Free exercise.
b. Assisted exercise.
c. Assisted- resisted exercise.
d. Resisted exercise.

B. *Involuntary movement : Reflex movement*

2. Passive Movement

A. *Relaxed passive movements.*

B. *Passive manual mobilization techniques.*

a. Mobilisation of joints.
b. Manipulation of joints.
c. Controlled sustained stretching .

Active Movement

Voluntary Movement

Movement performed or controlled by the voluntary action of muscles, working in opposition to an external force or we can say movement which is performed by the patient voluntarily.

CLASSIFICATION

- Free Movement
- Assisted Movement

- Assisted – resisted Movement
- Resisted Movement

FREE MOVEMENT

Free movements are those which are performed by the patient's own muscular efforts without the assistance or resistance of any external force, other than that of gravity. They vary widely in character and effect, not only because of the nature and extent of the movement but according to the manner in which they are performed.

Advantage

The great advantage of free exercise is home practice. To help the patient largely depends on his desire for rehabilitation and his confidence in the efficiency of the exercise

Disadvantages

Patient's with neuromuscular disorder require more redevelopment or reinforcement of weak muscles. When there is muscular imbalance compensatory rather than normal patterns of movement may be used unless movements are carefully taught and supervised. Patients need to be cooperative in doing these exercises until their performance has been facilitated and voluntary control has been established

Classification

1. *Localized movement*

Designed primarily to produce some local and specific effect, for example, to mobilize a particular joint or to strengthen particular muscle groups, Movement is localized to one or more joints, either by the use of a suitable starting position, or by voluntary fixation of other areas by the patient's own muscular efforts.

2. *Generalized movement*

Usually involve the use of many joints and muscles all over the body and the effects are widespread, for example as in running.

3. Subjective movement

Exercises which are subjective are usually formal and consist of more or less anatomical movements performed in full range The attention of the patient is deliberately focused on the form and pattern of the exercise to ensure accuracy of performance

4. Objective movement

Objective movement are those during the performance of which the patient attention is concentrated on the achievement of a particular aim which will result his efforts e.g. standing - Arm stretching upwards, to touch a mark on the wall.

Prerequisites for Free Movements

The Starting Position

Interest and cooperation of the patient lead him to understand both the pattern and the purpose of the exercise.

- Speed of the exercise
- Duration of the exercise

The Effects and Uses

The effect and consequent uses of any particular free exercise depends on the exercise, its extent the intensity and duration of its performance

1. Relaxation

Rhythmical swinging movement and those which are pendular in character assist the relation of hypertonic muscles in the region of the joint moved. The alternating and reciprocal contractor and relaxation of the opposing muscles groups. This is required to sustain movement, help to restore the normal state of relaxation which follows contraction. This type of exercise is used in conjunction with other methods which induce relaxation of reduce a state of wasteful tension in muscles, which limits the range of joints movements and reduces the efficiency of neuromuscular coordination. Exercise which involve particular muscle groups strongly achieve reciprocal relaxation of the opposing muscle group e.g. work for the Scapular Retractors and shoulders extensors assist relaxation of the Pectoral Muscles.

2. Joint mobility

The normal joint movements are maintained by exercises of full range. If and when the range of movement is limited, the free range exercise many serve to increase it.

3. Muscle power and tone

The power and endurance of the working muscles are maintained or increased when the exercise is performed at any speed which is slower or rapid. Than when the natural speed of movement is employed, and it increases with the duration of the exercise, A high degree of tension and consequent increase on power can develop by free exercise when the muscles work for any time against the resistance offered by the body weight, or against the mechanical disadvantages of an leverage provided by a long and heavy limb. Normally, muscle power is maintained adequately by a minimum of everyday activities, most of which are performed in the middle range , Under abnormal conditions , however for example during fixation of a joint, the power can only be maintained or improved by repeated static contractor , which the patient must practice through out the days.

4. Neuromuscular coordination

Neuromuscular coordination is improved by the repetition of an exercise. As the pattern of movement is established it is simplified and becomes more efficient and the conduction of the necessary activities, in which at one time required concentration and efforts, become with practice more or less automatic in character, and skill is developed, as for example in walking or playing the piano.

5. Confidence

The achievement of coordinate and efficient movement assures the patient of his ability to maintain subjective control of his body, giving him confidence to attempt new activities, together with a feeling of exhilaration and satisfaction when they are accomplished. For example, jumping a rope or shooting a goal objective exercise and activities are usually used for this purpose

6. Circulatory and respiratory operation

During the vigorous of prolonged exercise it is apparent that the speed and depth of respiration is increased, that the heart beats faster and more forcefully and that heat is produced where as in light exercise the changes are so slight that they are nor notices.

ASSISTED MOVEMENT

When the force exerted on one of the body lever by muscular action as insufficient for the production or control of movement, an external force may be added to complete the movement. This external force must be applied in the direction of the muscle action but not necessary at the same point.

Prerequisite for Assisted Movement

- Starting Position
- Pattern of Movement
- Support
- The assisting force
- The range of movement
- The character of the movement
- Repetitions
- The co-operation of the patient

Effect and Uses of Assisted Movement

- The working muscles demand assisting force from the other muscles to gain in strength which is special type of exercise may be used in the early stages of neuromuscular reeducation.
- Assisted exercise frequently used in training and coordination of the affected muscle.
- Provide confidence for the painful joints as for example in Rheumatoid arthritis
- The range of effective joint movement may be increased by assisted exercise.

ASSISTED – RESISTED MOVEMENT

Active assisted - resisted movement is a type of exercise which constitutes a combination of assisted and resistance during a single movement and whenever it is possible, it is preferable to have assisted exercise as it meets the needs of the muscles with greater accuracy.

RESISTED MOVEMENT

Resisted movement is a part of exercise in which an external force may be applied to the body levers to oppose the force of muscular contraction. Tension is increased within the muscles by the opposing force (or resistance) and the muscles respond by an increase in this power and hypertrophy. The resisting force applied to an isotonic contraction must be sufficient to increase intra – muscular tension to the maximum without interfering with the ability of the muscles to produce coordinated movement.

Factors

Power, endurance, volume, speed of contraction and coordination are five factors which contribute the development of muscular efficiency out of which Power, endurance and volume can be built up by the use of resisted exercise.

Variation of the Power of Muscles on Different Parts of their Range

Muscles which are capable of producing a considerable range of joint movement do not equally power all through their range.

Physiologically muscles are capable of exerting their greatest strength when they are fully extended, e.g. in outer range and as they shorten their force diminishes. This however is modified some cases e.g. the effect of the pull on the lever is greatest when the angle of pull approaches a right angle. For example physiologically the flexors of the elbow are strongest in their outer range but technically strongest at about mid range when both these factors are taken into account and allowance is made for overcoming the initial inertia at the beginning of the movement, it can be roughly estimated that the muscles will be most efficient in the outer part of the middle range. This in fact can be proved by experiments.

It seems however, that the relative importance of these factors various in different muscle groups, but broadly speaking, each group is found to be most powerful in the part of the range in which it is habitually used i.e. shoulder flexors in outer range. Hip extensors in inner range. In giving manual resistance these variations in power can be felt and the resistance is adjusted accordingly, but other means of providing resistance are not so accurate from this point of view.

Prerequisite for Resisted Movement

- Starting Position
- Pattern of Movement
- Fixation
- Traction
- The resisting force
- The character of the movement
- Repetitions
- The co-operation of the patient

Resistances

Resisting force may be applied by various method on human body are as follows:

- The physiotherapist – This is usually applied manually in the line of the movement, and the physiotherapist's hand.
- The patient – The patient can resist his own movement with the sound limb or by using his own body weight.
- Weights – Weights is a simple and effective method of resisting active exercise in the form of sandbags or metal bags are used, a canvas bag may be strapped to the part and any number of units of weights can be inserted to provide the required resistance.
- Weights and pulley circuits – Rope and pulley may act as a resistance force during active muscular force generated by body.
- Spring and other elastic substance – The resistance force of a spring increase progressively as it is stretched or

compressed according to the type of spring used. Other extensible materials such as rubber elastic of various widths and thickness behave in a manner similar to that springs, but that are not so durable.

- Substance which are malleable—Substances such as putty clay , some kinds of wax, plasticine and weight sand can be moulded into different shapes, the resistance they offer to this change in the form is variable and can be used both for strengthening and for mobilizing the hands
- Water – Water can give resistance exercise during the limb movement inside the water against the buoyant force.

Type of resisted exercises

1. Isotonic resistance exercise
2. Isometric resistance exercise
3. Isokinetic resistance exercise

PROGRESSIVE RESISTED EXERCISE (PRE)

Progressive resistance exercise was developed by De Lorme for the restoration of muscle power and volume after injury in 1945. Metal weight, which constitute the resisting force, are applied to the part of the body in question either by means of a bar bell held in the hand or hands, a de lorme metal boot or some similar device. The poundage is determined by testing the repetition. Lifting of the weight may involve either static (isometric) or dynamic (isotonic) muscle work according to the circumstances and the movement is slow and controlled. Several way of correlating the weight lifted and the number of repetition has been used. It appears that the regime most suitable and successful in the treatment of an individual patient varies very much with this age, temperament and the conditions from which he is suffering, it is essential that his instructions are precise and that his efforts are well supervised. The following schemes are all based on the test for a 10 R.M. and represent a power programme. Internal measures can be replaced by metric units. The endurance programme is based on the use of relatively low resistance and high repetition regime. Progressive exercise can be used in principle for the development of most muscles group but it is at present more often used for the knee Extensors that any other groups. Some suggestion with regards to suitable position and methods are therefore described in relation to these muscles.

Repetition maximum (RM)

It is used in PRE to measure the strengthed of the given muscle, so that the muscle can be strengthen onwards to its maximum strength. e.g.- One RM is the maximum amount of resistance or load that can be lifted only once through available range of motion. Two RM is the maximum amount of resistance or load that can be lifted twice through available range of motion. 10 RM is the maximum amount of resistance or load that can be lifted 10 times through available range of motion.

Progression

The apparatus used for assessment of R.M. is Quadriceps table, De Lorme Boot and straps. As the power of the muscle increases, the resistance must be increased proportionally. 'There are four main method of increasing resistance to muscle action. Each method may be used singly or in combination with any other method

- Increase in poundage or weight of the resisting force
- Increase in leverage of the resisting force
- Alteration in the speed of movement
- Increase in the duration of the exercise

Increase in Poundage or weight of the resisting force - For example: it is found that a muscle group, able to achieve full range contraction against a weight of 2 kg when it is supplied at a specific point, can contract at a specific weight is increased proportionally to 2 – 5 kg, 3 kg, 4 Kg while the other conditions remain constant.

The following schemes are generally used in daily clinical practice by the therapist and trainers.

1. **Oxford Technique (Zinovief)**

- 10 lifts with 10 RM
- 10 lifts with 10 RM minus 1 lb

- 10 lifts with 10 RM minus 2 lb
- 10 lifts with 10 RM minus 3 lb
- 10 lifts with 10 RM minus 4 lb
- 10 lifts with 10 RM minus 5 lb
- 10 lifts with 10 RM minus 6 lb
- 10 lifts with 10 RM minus 7 lb
- 10 lifts with 10 RM minus 8 lb
- 10 lifts with 10 RM minus 9 lb
- 100 lift for five times in a week progress, 10 RM daily

Every 10 lifts / repetitions are followed by brief period of rest.

2. De Lorme and Watkins

- 10 lifts with ½ 10 RM
- 10 lifts with ¾ 10 RM
- 10 lifts with full 10 RM
- 30 lift for 4 times a week, progress 10 RM once weekly. Every 10 repetition.

3. MacQueen

- 10 lifts with 10 RM
- 10 lifts with 10 RM
- 10 lifts with 10 RM
- 10 lifts with 10 RM
- 40 lifts for 3 times a week.

Progress 10 RM after every 1-2 weeks.

Active Movements of Upper Limb and Lower Limbs

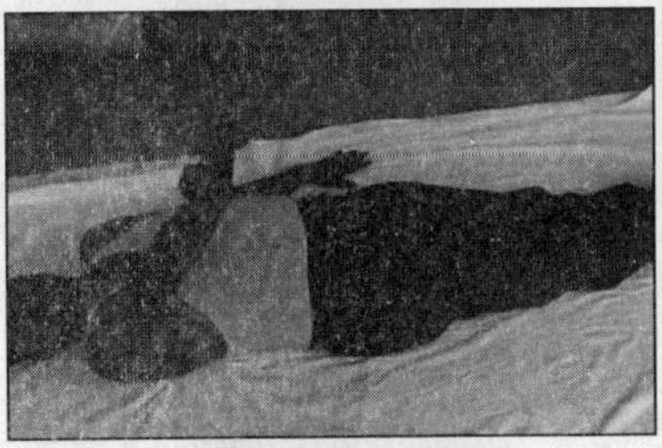

Fig. 16.1: *Shoulder flexion*

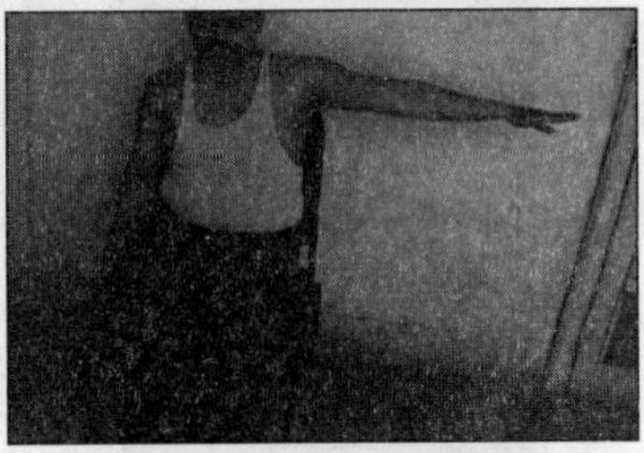

Fig 16.2: *Shoulder abduction*

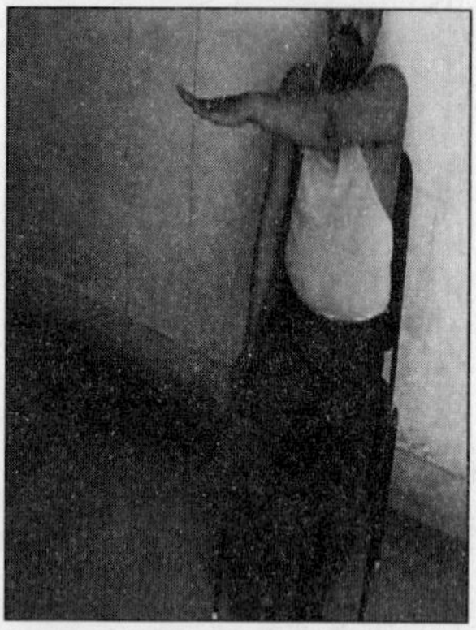

Fig. 16.3: *Shoulder horizontal adduction*

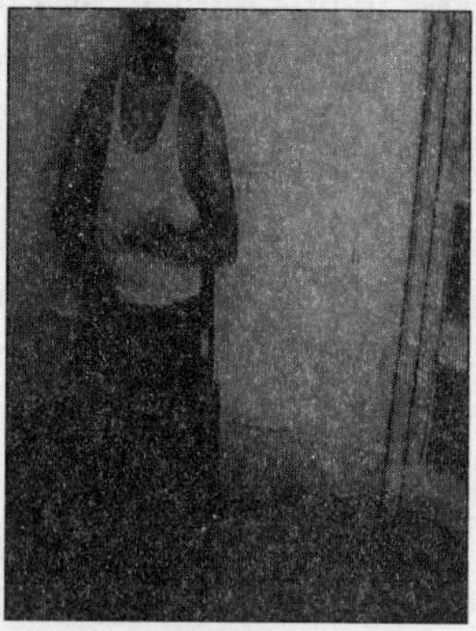

Fig. 16.4: *Shoulder internal rotation*

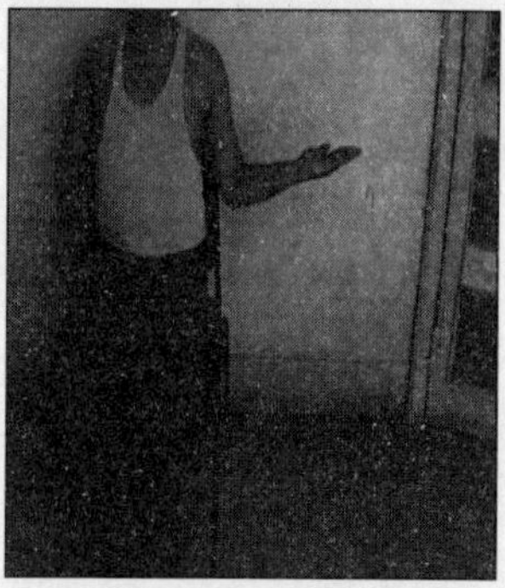

Fig. 16.5: *Shoulder external rotation*

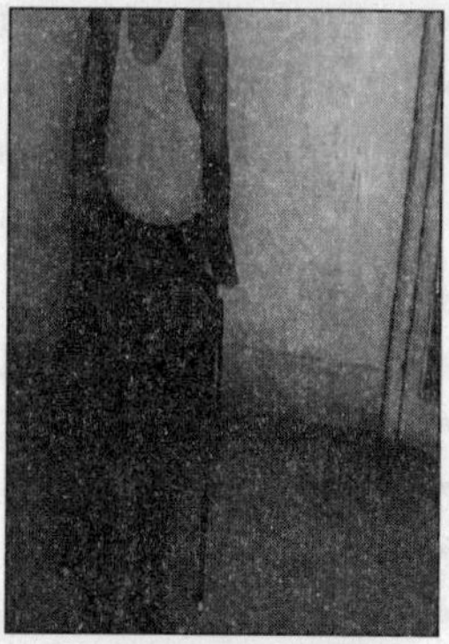

Fig. 16.6: *Forearm pronation*

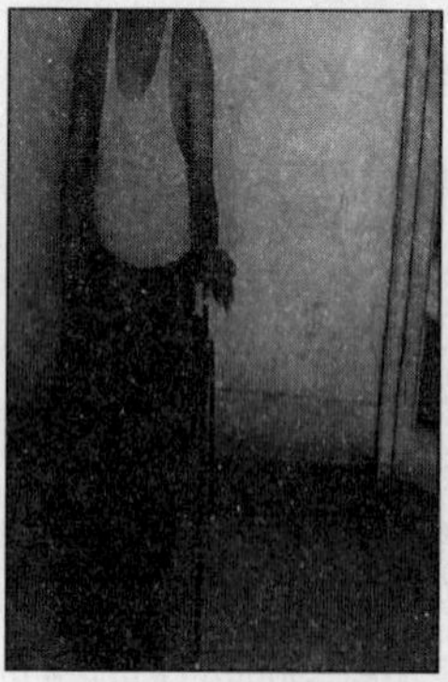

Fig. 16.7: *Forearm supination*

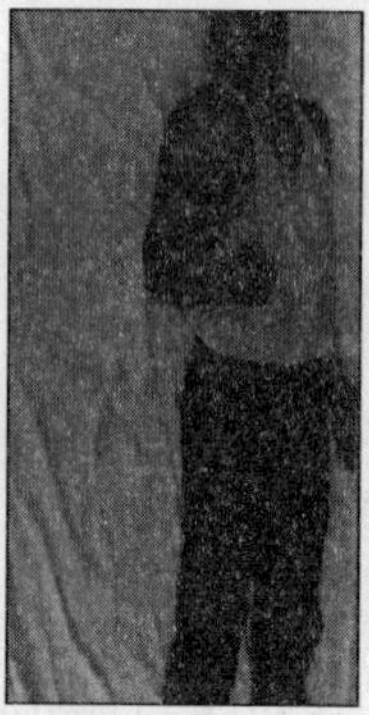

Fig. 16.8: *Elbow flexion*

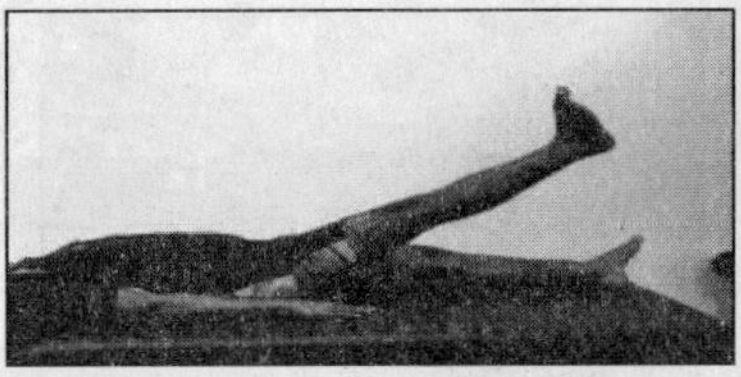

Fig. 16.9: *Hip flexion with knee extension*

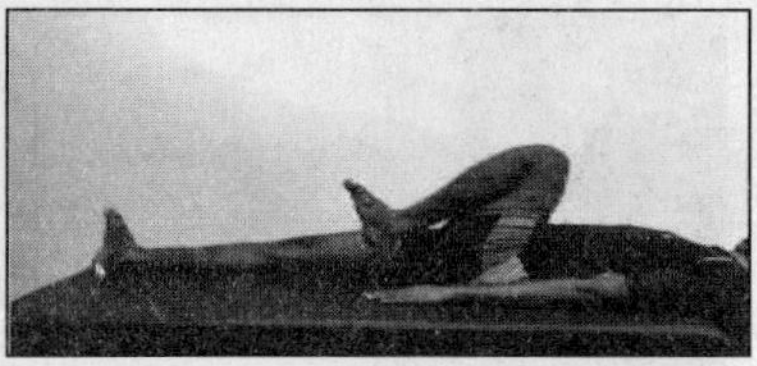

Fig. 16.10: *Hip flexion with knee flexion*

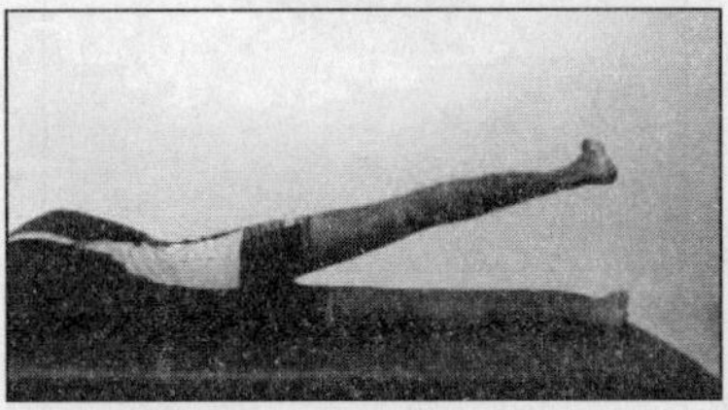

Fig.16.11: *Hip abduction*

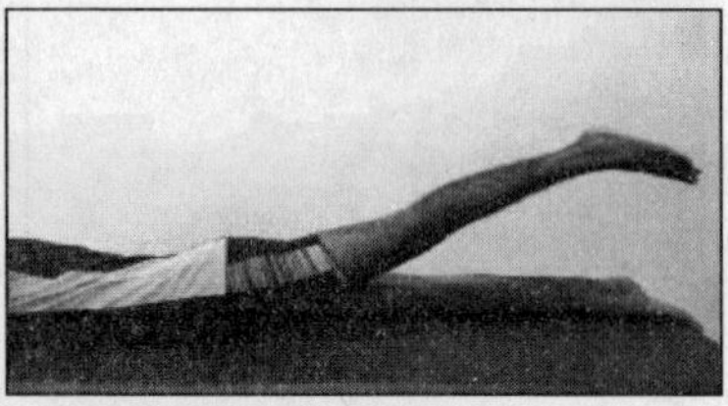

Fig. 16.12: *Hip hyperextension*

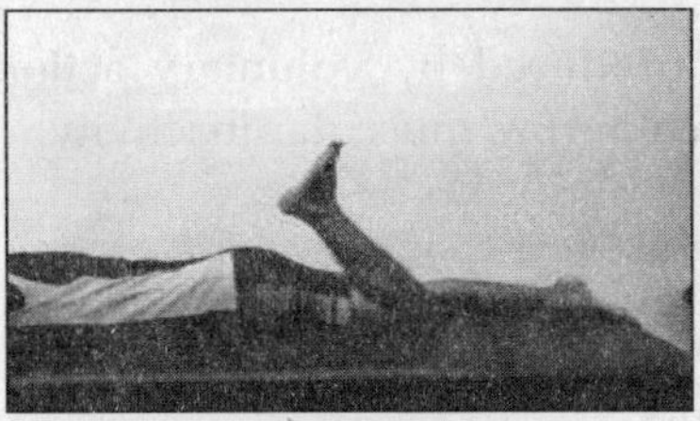

Fig. 16.13: *Knee flexion*

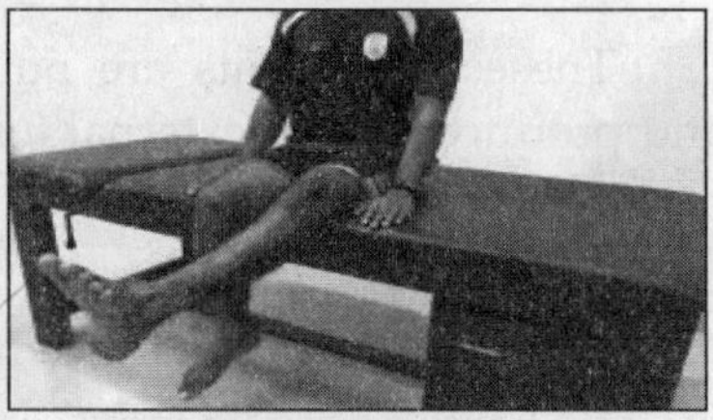

Fig. 16.14: *Knee extension*

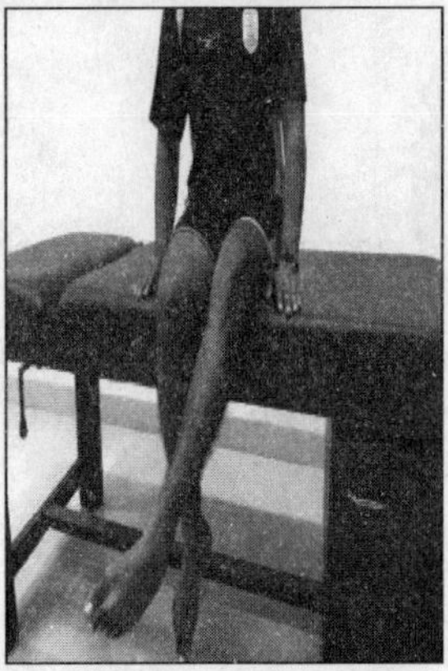

Fig. 16.15: *Hip external rotation*

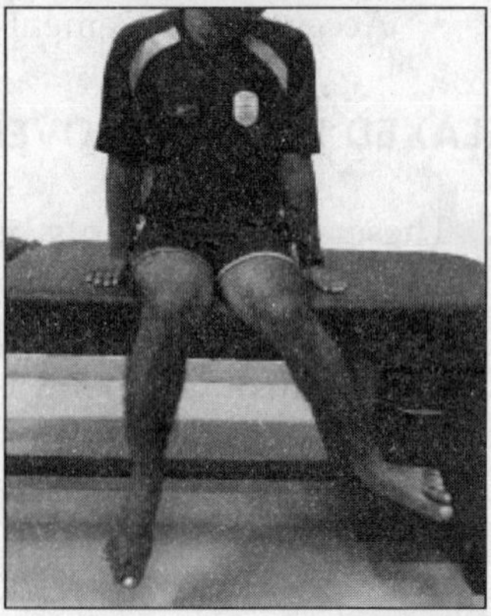

Fig. 16.16: *Hip internal rotation*

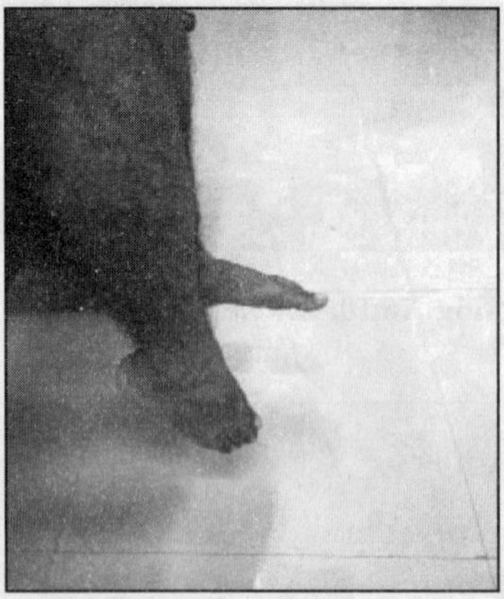

Fig. 16.17: *Ankle planter flexion*

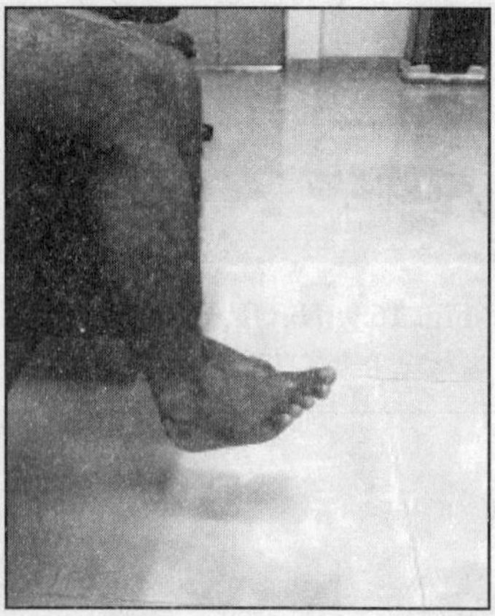

Fig. 16.18: *Ankle dorsiflexion*

PASSIVE MOVEMENT

These movements are not produced by voluntary action and produced by an external force during muscular inactivity.

TYPES

- Relaxed passive movement
- Forced passive movement
- Passive mobilization / manipulation techniques
- Accessory movement

RELAXED PASSIVE MOVEMENT

These are movements performed accurately and smoothly by physiotherapist. Knowledge of anatomy is required. The movements are performed in the same range and direction as active movement. The joint is moved through the existing free range and within pain free part of ROM.

Relaxed Passive Movements for Upper Limb and Lower Limbs

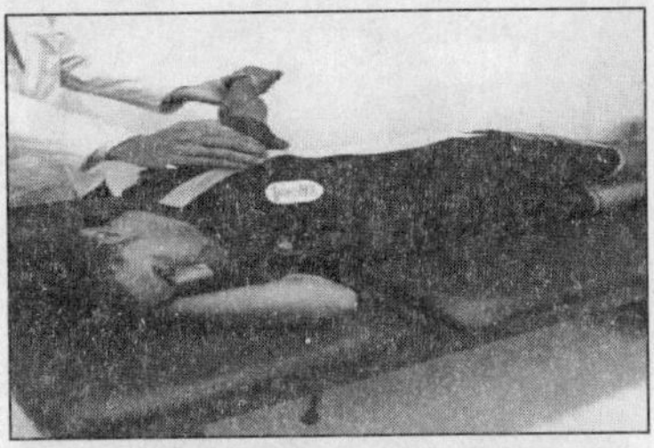

Fig. 16.19: *Shoulder extension*

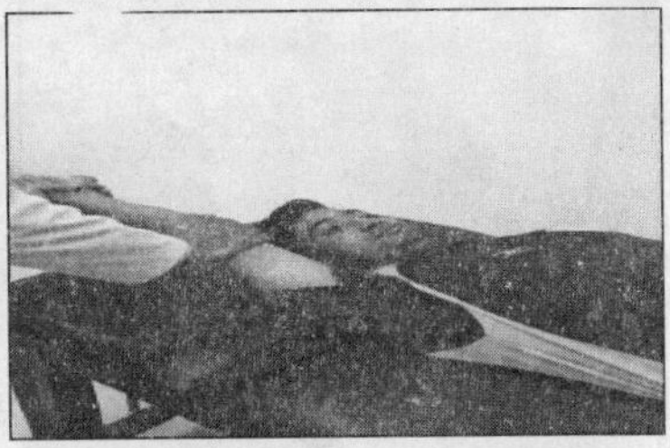

Fig. 16.20: *Shoulder flexion*

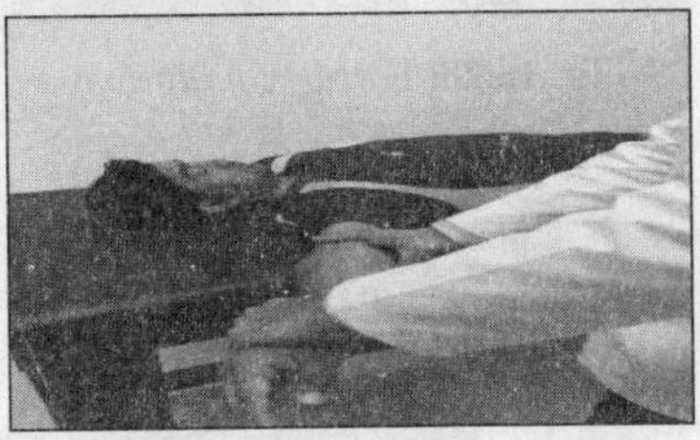

Fig 16.21: *Shoulder abduction*

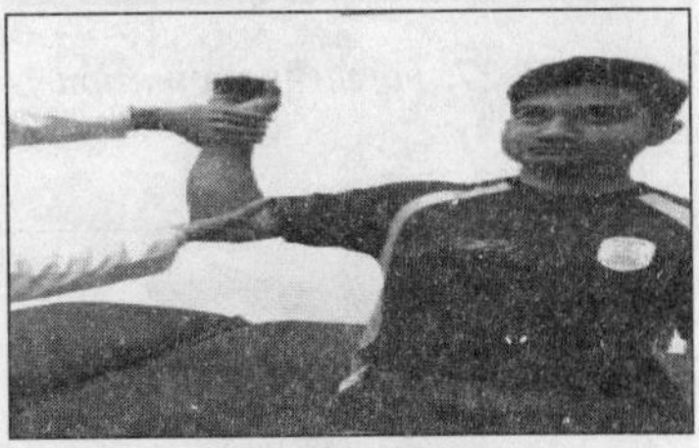

Fig 16.22: *Shoulder external rotation*

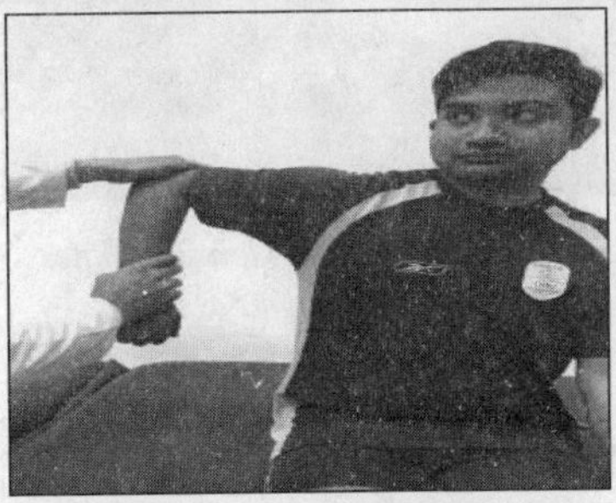

Fig. 16.23: *Shoulder medial rotation*

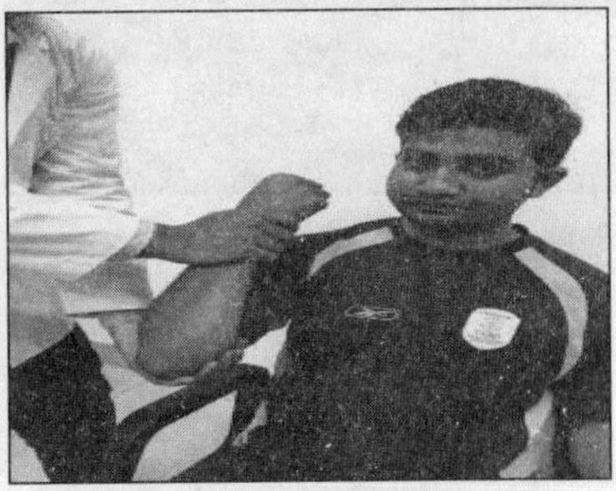

Fig. 16.24: *Elbow flexion*

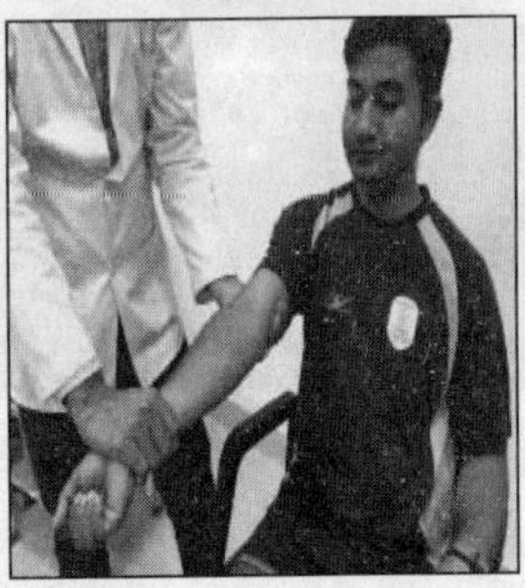

Fig. 16.25: *Elbow extension*

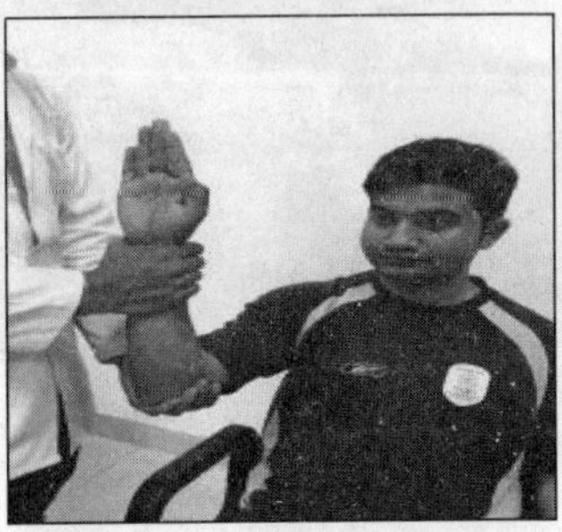

Fig. 16.26: *Forearm pronation*

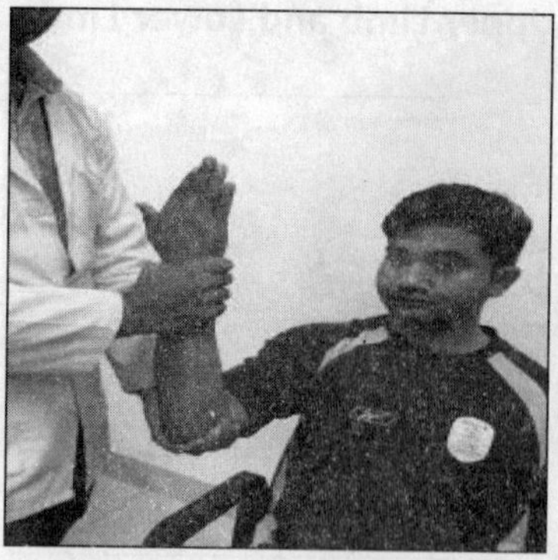

Fig. 16.27: *Forearm supination*

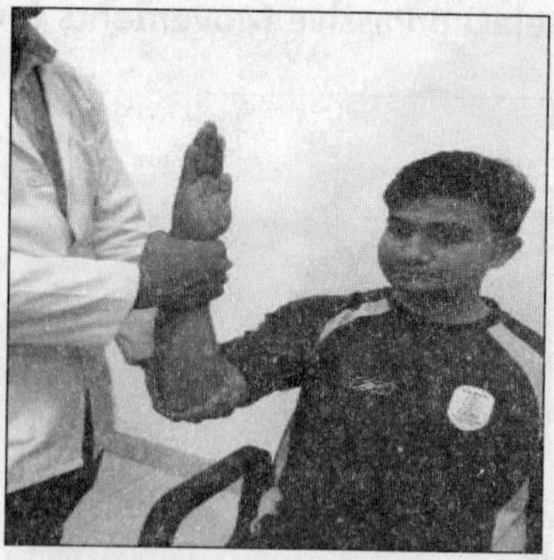

Fig. 16.28: *Forearm midprone*

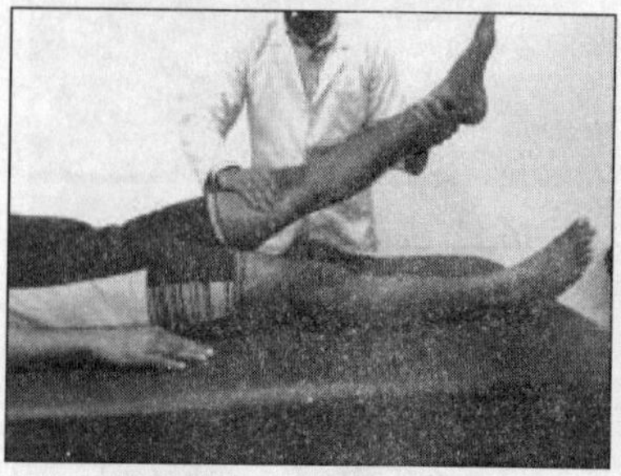

Fig. 16.29: *Hip flexion with knee extension*

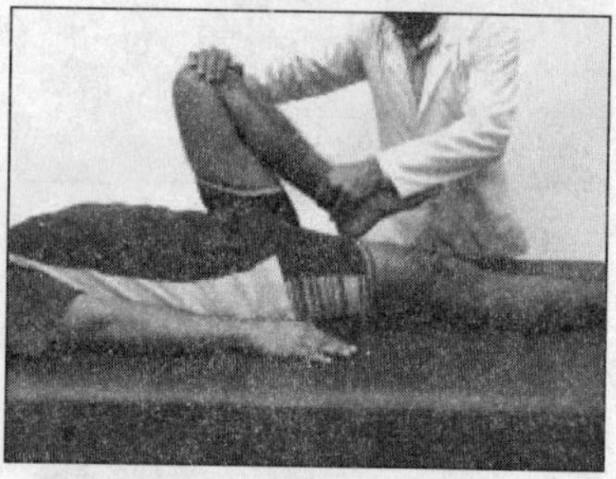

Fig. 16.30: *Hip flexion with knee flexion*

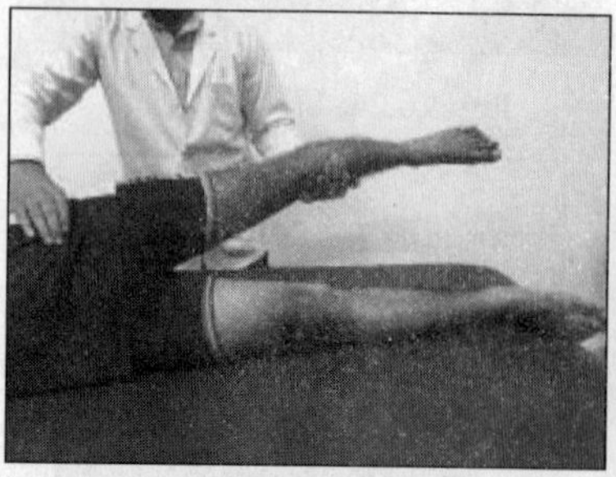

Fig. 16.31: *Hip hyperextension*

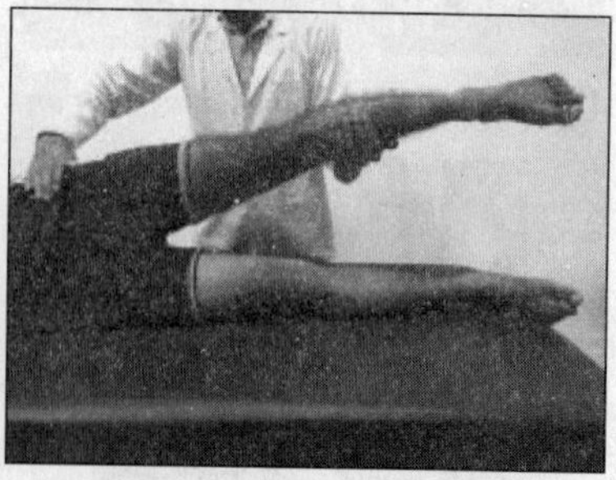

Fig. 16.32: *Hip abduction*

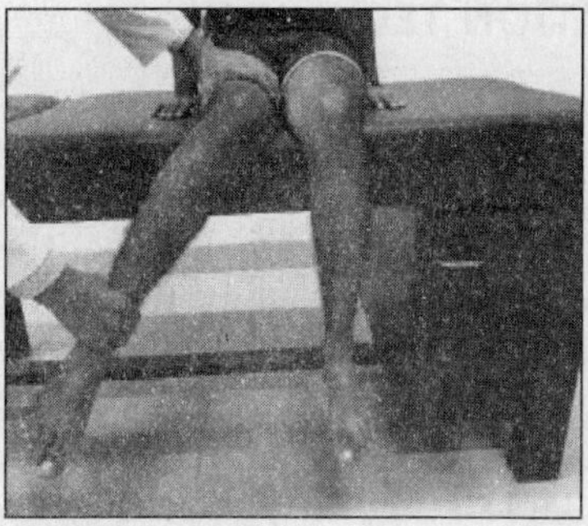

Fig. 16.33: *Hip internal rotation*

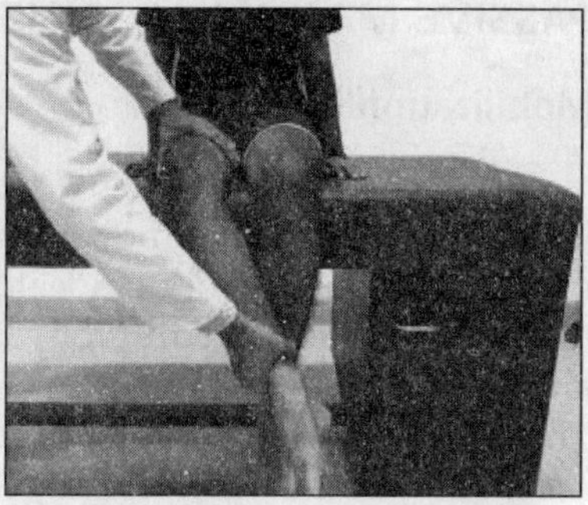

Fig. 16.34: *Hip external rotation*

Effects and Uses of Relaxed Passive Movement

Adhesions formation is prevented and the present free range of movement maintained

When active movement is impossible because of muscular inefficiency, these movements may help to preserve the memory of movement patterns by stimulating the receptors of kinesthetic sense

When full range of active movement is impossible and the extensibility of muscle is maintained and adaptive shortening is prevented.

The venous and lymphatic drainage may be assisted slightly by mechanical pressure and by stretching of the thin walled vessels which pass across the joint moved. Relatively quick, rhythmical and continued passive movements are required to produce this effect. They are used in conjunction with elevation of the part to relieve oedema, when the patient is unable or unwilling to perform sufficient active exercises

The rhythm of continued passive movement can have a soothing effect and induce further relaxation and sleep. They may be tried in training the patient for relaxation; if successful the movement is made imperceptibly and progressively slower as the patient relaxes.

PASSIVE MANUAL MOBILIZATION TECHNIQUE

Mobilization of Joints

A passive movement technique designed to improve joint function. These movements are usually small repetitive rhythmical oscillatory, localized accessory or functional movements performed by physiotherapist in various amplitude and within the available range and under the patient's control. These can be done very gently or quite strongly and are graded according to the part of the available range in which they are performed.

Grades of Movement

Grade 1 : Small amplitude movement performed at the beginning of range.

Grade 2 : Large amplitude movement performed with in the range, but not reaching the limit of the range and not returning to the beginning of range.

Grade 3 : Large amplitude movement performed upto the limit of range.

Grade 4 : Small amplitude movement performed at the limit of range.

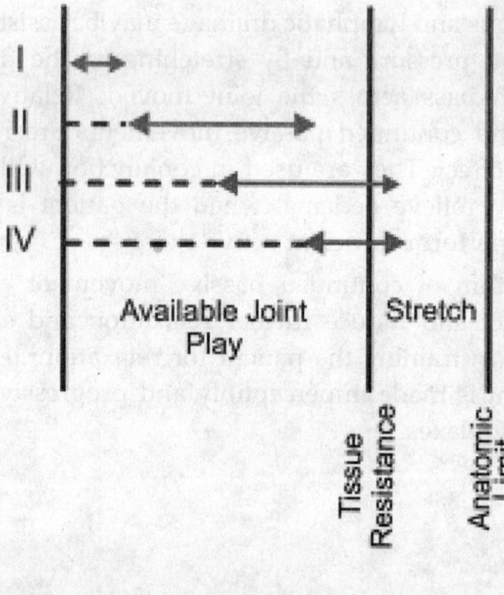

Mobilization Technique

- The patient should have a general understanding of the purpose of mobilization.
- The patient should be completely relaxed during treatment.
- The therapist should be in a comfortable position while performing mobilization activities.
- The therapist's position should allow for optimal control of movement.
- Explain specific mobilization techniques to the patient prior to beginning treatment.
- Complete a general examination of each patient prior to beginning mobilization activities.
- Use gravity to assist with mobilization whenever possible.
- Mobilization activities are usually performed initially with the joint in a loose packed position
- Maintain contact with the mobilizing hand as close to the joint space as possible.
- Allow one digit to palpate the joint line when possible.
- Mobilize one joint in one direction at a time.
- Use a mobilization belt or wedge to assist with stabilization when necessary.
- Constantly modify mobilization techniques based on individual patient response.
- Compare the quality and quantity of joint play bilaterally.
- Reassess each patient prior to each treatment session.
- Manipulation of joints performed by physiotherapist

These are accurately localized single. Quick decisive movement of small amplitude and high velocity completed before the patient can stop it.

- Manipulations of joints performed by surgeon / physician

The movements are performed under anesthesia by a surgeon / physician to gain further range. The increase in movement must be maintained by physiotherapist.

Controlled or Sustained Stretching of Tightened Structure

Passive stretching of muscles and other soft tissues can be given to increase range of movement. Movement can be gained by the stretching adhesions in these structures by lengthening of muscle due to inhibition of tendon protective reflex.

Effects and uses of Controlled or Sustained Stretching of Tightened Structure

Steady and sustained stretching may be used to overcome spasticity patterns of limbs, e.g. a hemiplegic patient. The slow stretch produces a relaxation and lengthening of muscle.

A steady and prolonged passive stretch can overcome the resistance of shortened ligaments, fascia and fibrous sheaths of muscles as for example in controlled stretching and progressive splintage of talipes equino varus.

ACCESSORY MOVEMENT

These occur as part of any normal joint movement but may be limited or absent in abnormal joint conditions. They consist of gliding or rotational movement which can't be performed in isolation as a voluntary movement but can be isolated by physiotherapist.

Effects and uses of Accessory Movement

Accessory movements contribute to the normal function of joint in which they take place or that of adjacent joints. In abnormal joint conditions there may be limitation of these movements due to loss of full active range caused by stiffness of joint from contractures of soft tissue, adhesion formation or muscular inefficiency. These movements are performed by the physiotherapist to increase the lost range of movement and to maintained joint mobility. Hence they form an important part of the treatment of a patient who is unable to perform normal active movement.

CONTRAINDICATIONS OF PASSIVE MOVEMENT

- Arthrosis
- Pulmonary embolism
- Open wounds
- Deep vein thrombosis

PHYSIOLOGICAL EFFECTS OF PASSIVE MOVEMENT

- Heat is produced below tissue
- Improved circulation.
- Breaking of adhesions.
- Increased and maintenance of joint range of motion.

■

(17)

HYDROTHERAPY

Hydrotherapy is defined as a procedure of using the Physical properties of water for the treatment of a patient. In Hydrotherapy water is used externally and only its physical properties are made use for treatment purpose. (Fig. 17.1)

PRINCIPLE OF HYDROTHERAPY

- Hydrotherapy must be given only by a qualified physiotherapist.
- The temperature of water should be maintained between 34 °C and 36.5°C (94°F and 96°F for hot water programme and not less than (60°F) for cold water programme.
- The hall containing the hydrotherapy pool should be well - ventilated but free of sudden cold breeze. Enough warm sheets and towels should be available for covering the body once the patients is out of pool. So as to prevent hypthermia.
- The pool and surrounding area must be cleaned with disinfectants.
- Code of dressing and hygiene must be observed strictly e.g. appropriate clothing should be made compulsory.
- The patient should be positioned appropriately so as to make the physical properties of water for facilitating exercises.

Hydrotherapy should be given only when it is prescribed with consideration to the age and conditions of the patient. It should not be given when contraindicated.

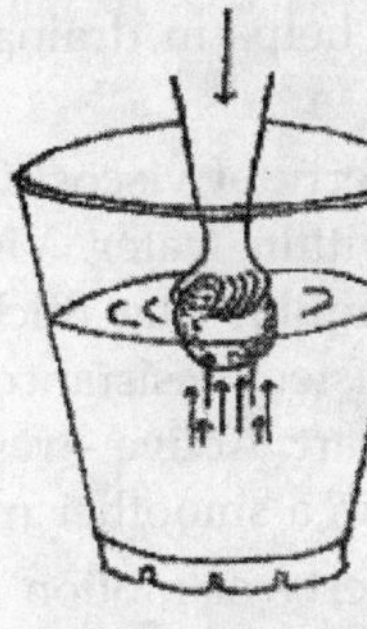

Fig: *17.1: Hydrotherapy*

EFFECTS OF HYDROTHERAPY

- Contact with cold water causes contraction of blood vessels and this contraction relieves congestion in the blood vessel.
- Contact with warm water causes dilation of blood vessels and this dilation increases blood supply.
- The physical property of buoyancy balances the force of gravity. 'Buoyancy is the upward thrust exerted by liquids on a body which is submerged in that liquid. This upward thrust almost neutralizes the force of gravity. Thus the person experiences a relief in its own weight as well as relief from the pull of gravity'. Active - free movements can therefore be done with minimum efforts in water.
- Buoyancy helps the body to float horizontally or vertically. It does not have turning effects on the body so the body can take up required body position much easily in the waterpool than in a gymnasium.
- The physical property of hydrostatic pressure causes equal pressure to be exerted in all directions on the submerged limb. Hydrostatic pressure is the pressure exerted by water on its container and contents submerged in it when the water is at rest. Water like any other liquid, exerts different pressures when in motion. This equi- directional pressure acts like a gentle and consistence light massage. A gentle and squeezing action

takes place which helps in drainage of excessive tissue fluids.

- The physical property of viscosity offers a resistance to limb movement within water. Viscosity is thickness of consistency of a liquid. The thick consistence offers a constant and consistent resistance to any movement of submerged body part. Active – resistive movements can therefore be done in a smoother manner in water.
- The physical property of motion of the water offers an external force. This force in the form of water currents used as an assistive force or a resistance force by positioning the limb and body appropriately in the direction or against the direction of the current respectively. Active assistive and active – resistive movements respectively can therefore be achieved in a smoother manner with the help of these currents and helps in keeping the person healthy. It has medical applications for persons with skin conditions, physiotherapeutic hydrotherapy for persons having musculoskeletal problems.

TYPES OF HYDROTHERAPY

1. Fitness activities for healthy person.
2. Medical applications for persons with skin conditions.
3. Physiotherapeutic Hydrotherapy for persons having musculoskeletal problems.

Note: Here, attention is paid only to the physiotherapeutic hydrotherapy type.

Physiotherapeutic Hydrotherapy

In physiotherapeutic type of hydrotherapy emphasis is given to movements and exercises in the pool of water. Such a programme is also referred to as Pool exercises. This type of hydrotherapy is carried out in purpose built similar to a swimming pool. Most pool having static water is used. At times pools with artificially created motions of water called, whirlpools are used. Cold water baths are also used. A session of hydrotherapy lasts from 5 minutes to 30 minutes. Physiotherapeutic hydrotherapy has the following purposes as-

- Subsides swelling (cold water)
- Reduces inflammation and relieves pain
- Relieves spasm in the muscle and induces relaxation, thus increasing efficiency of contraction in the muscle
- Increases tone of the muscle
- Increases power of the muscle
- Increases range of motion in joints
- Improves respiration and increases stamina

Indication

- Muscular problems
- Skeletal problems
- Poor motor developments
- General disability

Contraindication

- Cardiac conditions
- Respiratory conditions
- Renal conditions including in continence
- Vascular conditions
- Open wounds
- Convulsions
- Menstruation
- Recent skin grafting

Whirlpool Bath

Whirlpool therapy is a combination of massage and water immersion. It has become one of the most popular thermotherapy used in sports medicine. The whirlpool is basically a tank and a turbine motor, which regulates the movement of water and air. (Fig. 17.2) The amount of movement is controlled by the amount of air that is emitted. There are three types of whirlpools are as-

1. *The extremity tank*—It is used for treating legs and arms and is 15 inches wide, 28-32 inches long, and 18-25 inches deep.
2. *The lowboy tank*—It is 24 inches wide, 52 – 62 inches long and 18 inches deep and is used for full body immersion.

3. *Highboy tank*—It is designed for the hip and leg and is 20 - 24 inches wide, 36 - 48 inches long and 28 inches deep.

Indication

The whirlpool provides both conduction and convection. Conduction is achieved by the skin's contact with the higher water temperature. As water swirls around the skin surface, convection occurs.

Application

The temperature should be set according to the condition. Once the tank has been filled with water at the desired temperature, the person is comfortably positioned so that the part to be treated can be easily reached by the agitated water. Treatment time should be increased slowly on a daily basis to 5 minutes, 10 minutes, 15 minutes and finally 20 minutes. Duration of 20 minutes is usually recommended for treatment of chronic injuries.

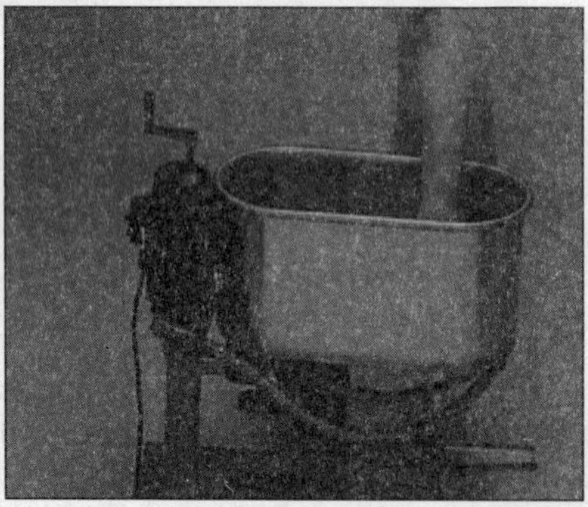

Fig: *17.2: Massage in hand through whirlpool bath*

BUTTERFLY BATH

The butterfly bath is charecterised by its practicle, ergonomic shape. (Fig. 17.3) The shape and dimensions of the butterfly bath allow various arm and leg exercises to be carreid out without heating the sides of the bath. The lift system can be lowered into the bath on a strecther. The bath can be provided with very strong under water jet massage unit.

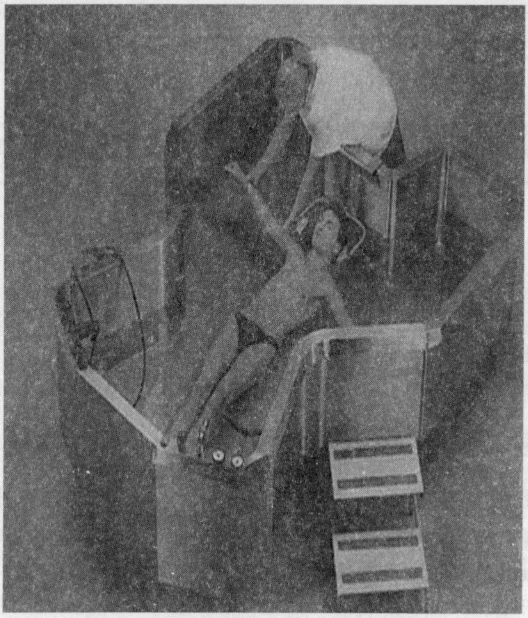

Fig: *17.3: Butterfly bath*

18

THERAPEUTIC EXERCISES

FLEXIBILITY EXERCISES

Flexibility is the range of movement possible at a specific joint or series of articulation. It is the general absence of stiffness.

Two Types

Static Flexibility—Refers to the amount of movement obtained by passively moving a limb to a maximum degree.

Dynamic Flexibility—Refers to the amount of active movement possible as a result of muscle contraction.

Effect of Flexibility Exercises

Two major importance of flexibility training i.e. performance enhancement and injury prevention.

Performance Enhancement

To achieve maximum performance, a limb must be able to move through a non restricted range of motion. A limited range of movement can reduce work efficiency in these situations, however if flexibility is increased, force may be applied over an increased distance thus facilitating the performance.

Injury Prevention

Flexibility exercises may condition muscles, ligaments, and fascia to greater tensile strength and elasticity, leading to injury prevention. When a muscle is stretched, elongation is detected by the muscle spindle afferent nerve fibers. These receptors send impulses to the dorsal roots of spinal cord, causing a reflex which contracts the extrafusal fibers of the same muscle, in opposition to the original stretching force.

Technique of Flexibility

Static Stretching—Slowly and passively stretching the muscle to full range, and maintaining this stretched position with constant tension.

Ballistic—rapid jerking actions at end of range to force the tissues to stretch

Contract relax—isometrically contracting the stretched muscle, and then relaxing and passively stretching the muscle still further. This action is usually performed by a partner.

Contract-relax-agonist-contract—the same as contract relax, except that during the final stages of the stretching phase the muscle opposite the one being stretched is contracted.

Stretching exercises for trunk, upper limb and lower limb.

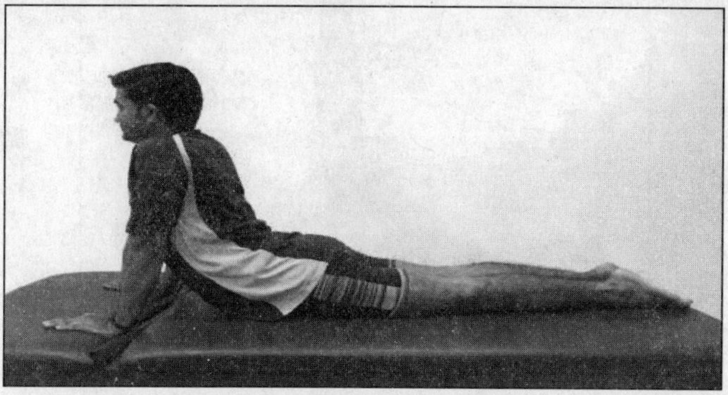

Fig. 18.1: *Stretching exercises for spine*

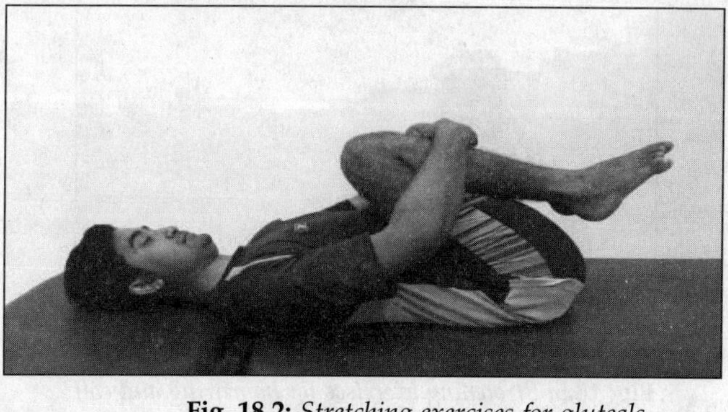

Fig. 18.2: *Stretching exercises for gluteals*

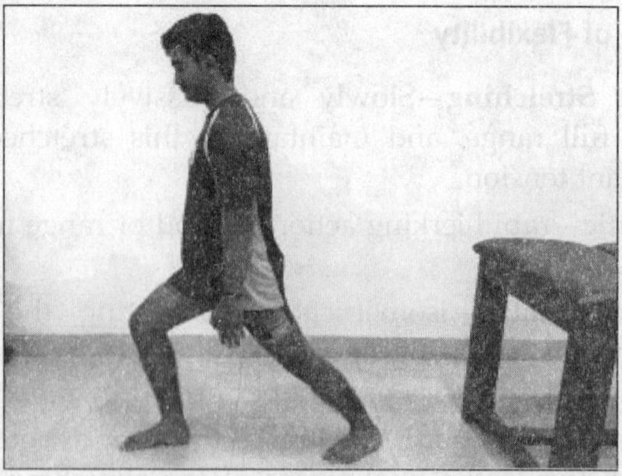

Fig. 18.3: *Stretching exercises for hip flexor*

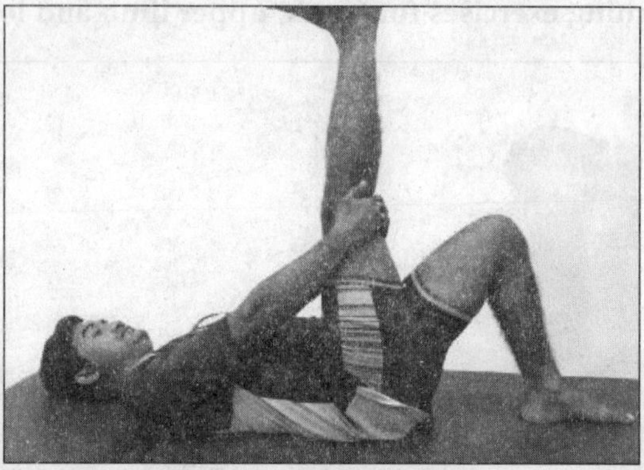

Fig. 18.4: *Stretching exercises for hamstring*

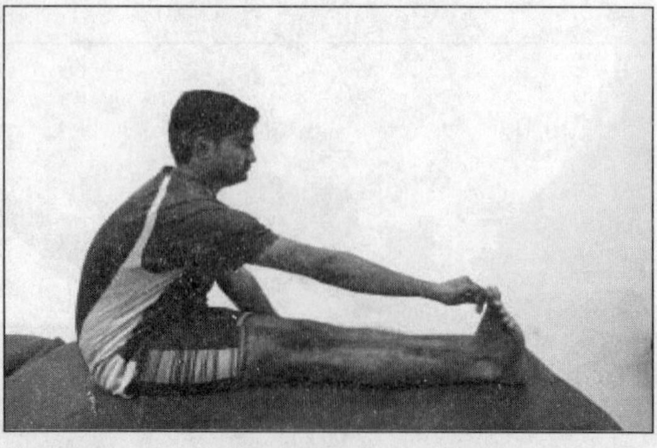

Fig. 18.5: *Stretching exercises for hamstring and calf*

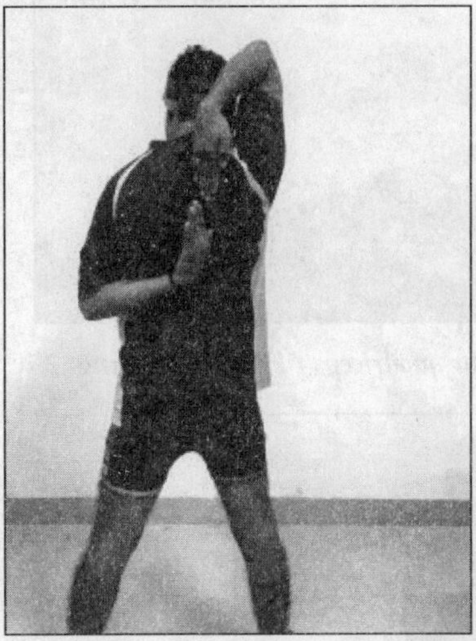

Fig. 18.6: *Stretching exercises for shoulder rotators*

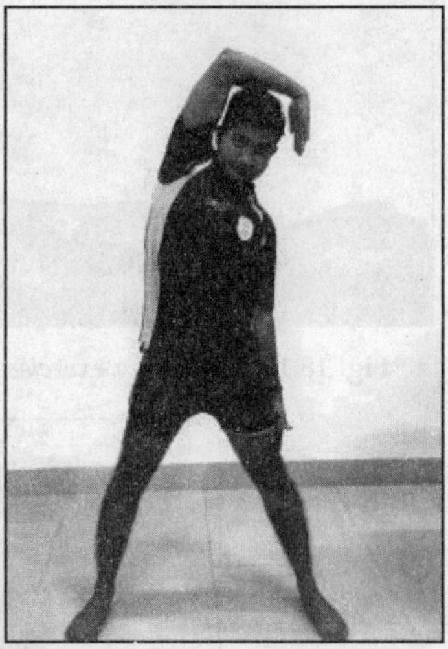

Fig. 18.7: *Stretching exercises for lateral trunk flexors*

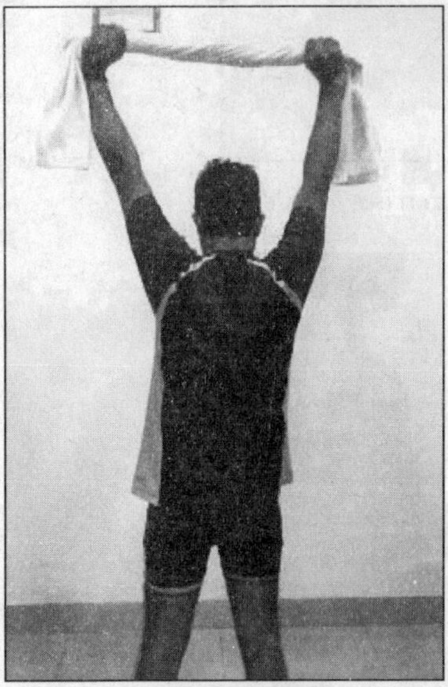

Fig. 18.8: *Stretching exercises for shoulder*

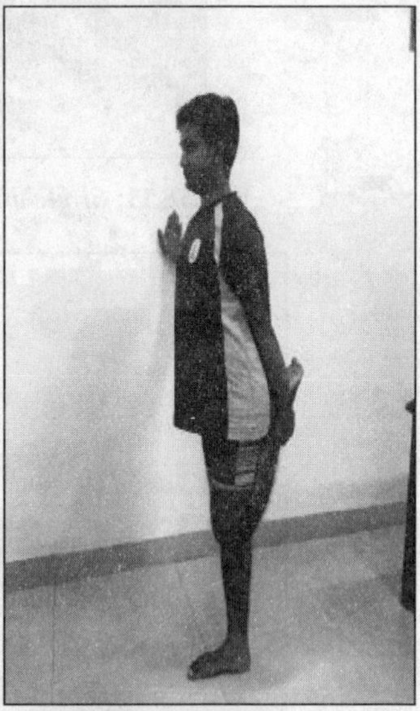

Fig. 18.9: *Stretching exercises for quadriceps / Hip flexors standing*

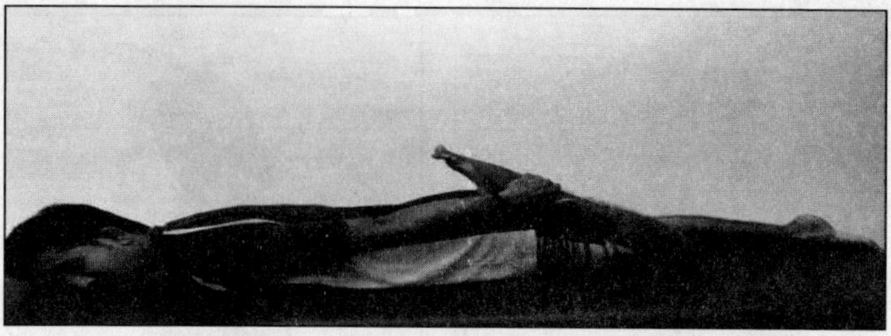

Fig. 18.10: *Stretching exercises for quadriceps / Hip flexors lying*

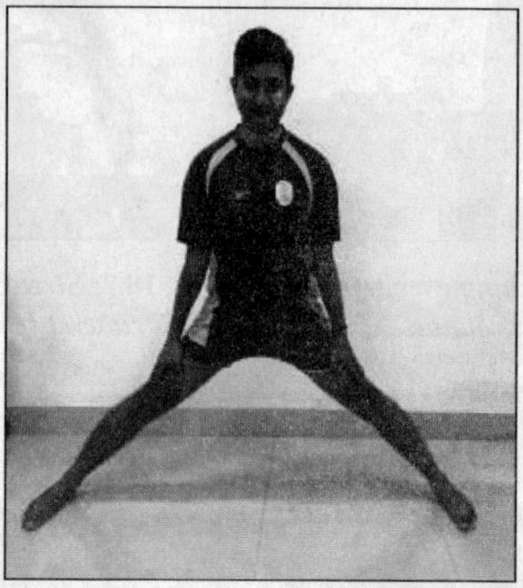

Fig. 18.11: *Stretching exercises for adductors*

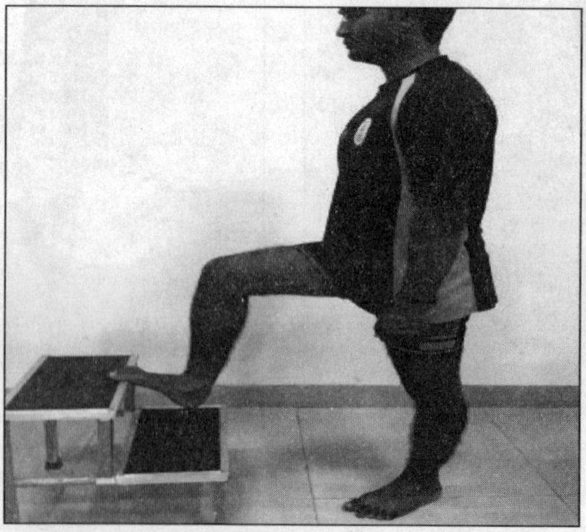

Fig. 18.12: *Self Stretching of planter flexor (Soleus)*

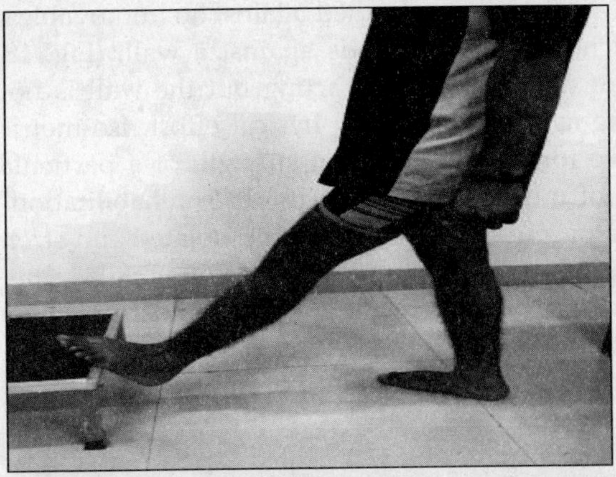

Fig. 18.13: *Self stretching of planter flexor (Gastrosoleus)*

Factors Affecting Flexibility: The external factors are temperature and the internal factors are muscle tissue, tendons, Joint capsule, bony contours etc.

STRENGTHENING EXERCISE

Strengthening exercise increases muscle strength and mass, bone strength, and the body's metabolism. It can help attain and maintain proper weight and improve body image and self-esteem. A certain level of muscle strength is needed to do daily activities, such as walking, running and climbing stairs. Strengthening exercises increase muscle strength by putting more strain on a muscle than it is normally accustomed to receiving. This increased load stimulates the growth of proteins inside each muscle cell that allow the muscle as a whole to contract. Weight training allows one to get immediate feedback, through observation of progress in muscle growth and improved muscle tone. Strengthening exercise can take the form of isometric, isotonic and iso-kinetic strengthening.

ISOMETRIC EXERCISE

During isometric exercises, muscles contract. However, there is no motion in the affected joints. The muscle fibers maintain a constant length throughout the entire contraction. The exercises are usually performed against an immovable surface or object such as pressing hands against a wall. (Fig. 18.14) The muscles of the arm are contracting but the wall is not reacting or moving as a result of the physical effort. Iso-metric training is effective for developing total strength of a particular muscle or group of muscles. It is often used for rehabilitation since the exact area of muscle weakness can be isolated and strengthening can be administered at the proper joint angle. This kind of training can provide a relatively quick and convenient method for overloading and strengthening muscles without any special equipment and with little chance of injury.

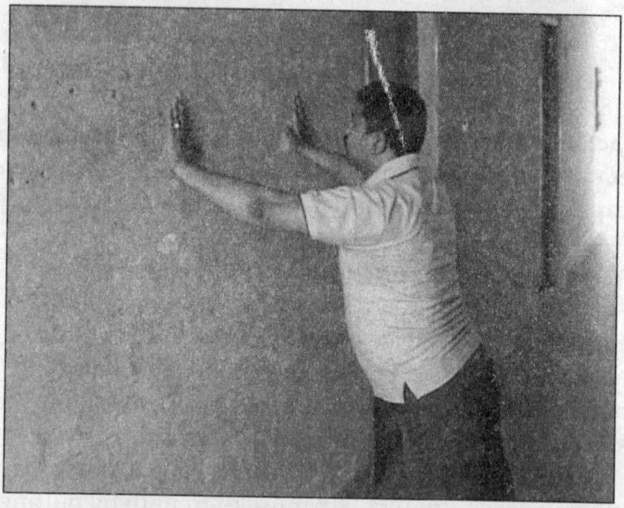

Fig. 18.14: *Isometric exercises to strengthen Upper limb*

ISOTONIC EXERCISE

Isotonic exercise differs from isometric exercise in that there is movement of a joint during the muscle contraction. A classic example of an isotonic exercise is weight training with dumbbells and barbells. (Fig. 18.15) As the weight is lifted throughout the range of motion, the muscle shortens and lengthens. Calisthenics are also an example of isotonic exercise. These would include chin-ups, push-ups, and sit-ups, all of which use body weight as the resistance force.

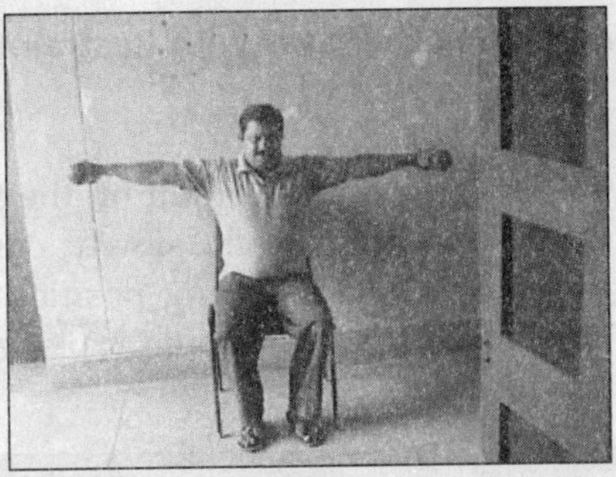

Fig. 18.15: *Isotonic exercises to strengthen upper limb*

ISOKINETIC EXERCISE

Isokinetic exercise utilizes machines that control the speed of contraction within the range of motion. Isokinetic exercise attempts to combine the best features of both isometrics and weight training. It provides muscular overload at a constant preset speed while a muscle mobilizes its force through the full range of motion. For example, an isokinetic stationary bicycle (Fig. 18.16) set at 90 revolutions per minute means that despite how hard and fast the exerciser works, the isokinetic properties of the bicycle will allow the exerciser to pedal only as fast as 90 revolutions per minute. Machines known as Cybex and Biodex provide isokinetic results; they are generally used by physical therapists and are not readily available to the general population.

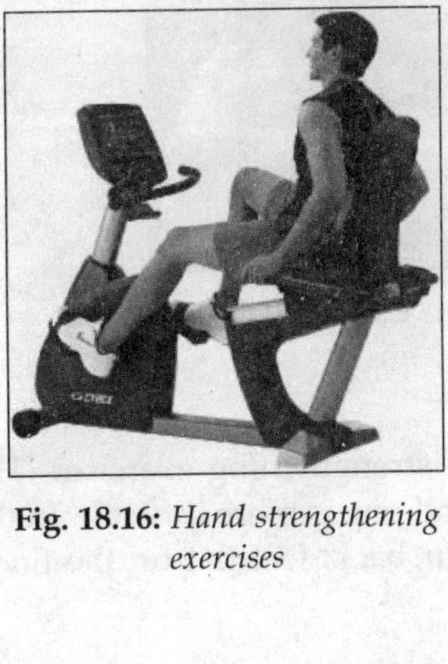

Fig. 18.16: *Hand strengthening exercises*

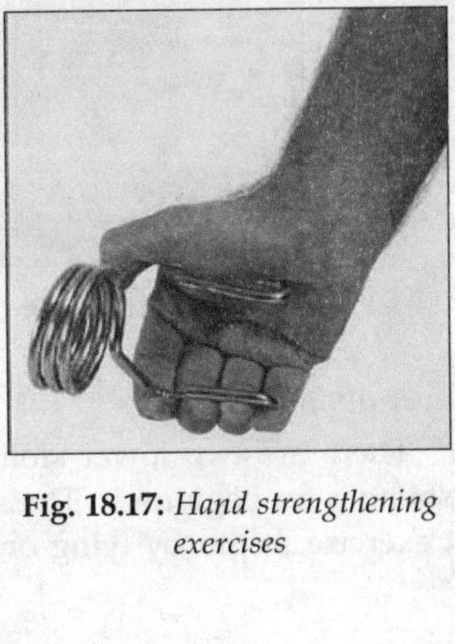

Fig. 18.17: *Hand strengthening exercises*

Approach Strengthening Exercises with Restraint (Fig. 18.17)

Curl ups

Start by lying on your back, feet flat on the floor. Keeping hands clasped and supporting neck, slowly curl upper body off the floor and then return to starting position. (Fig. 18.18) If possible, lift high enough to bring shoulder blades off the floor. Repeat until fatigued.

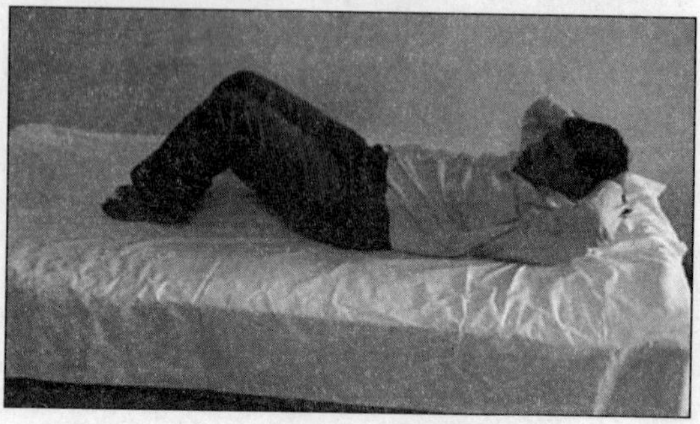

Fig. 18.18: *Curl ups*

Oblique Curl ups

Start by lying on your back, feet flat on the floor. Roll knees to one side. Do curl ups as above. Repeat until fatigued. (Fig. 18.19)

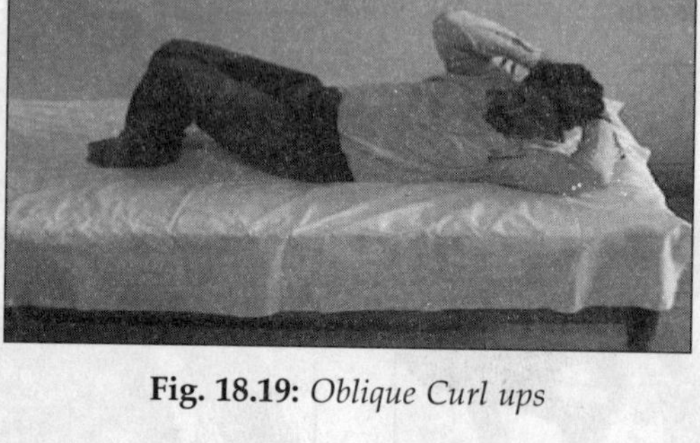

Fig. 18.19: *Oblique Curl ups*

Lower abdominals

There are two lower stomach strengthening exercises. The first one is for beginners. The second one is more difficult. In the 1st exercise, begin by lying on your back, feet flat on the floor.

Bring one knee up, push hand into knee but don't let your leg move. (Fig. 18.20) Hold for 5 seconds. Repeat with opposite leg. Do 10-20 times for each leg. For the 2nd exercise, begin in same starting position. Tighten stomach muscles and press low back into the floor. (Fig. 18.21) Maintaining that position, bring legs up toward chest. Slowly lower one leg down as shown but don't touch the floor. Bring leg back up and repeat with other leg. It is to be done until one gets fatigue.

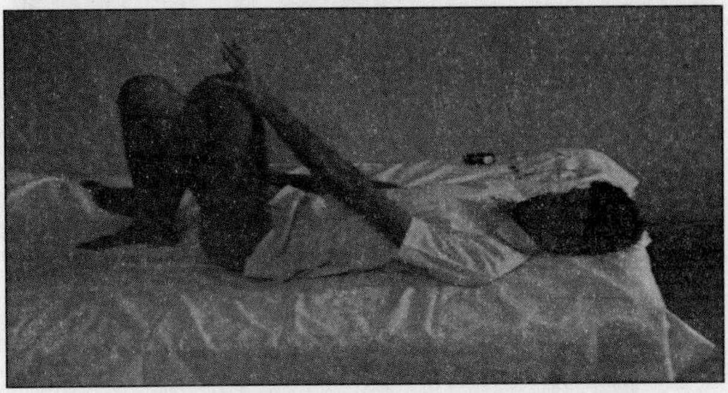

Fig. 18.20: *push hand into knee*

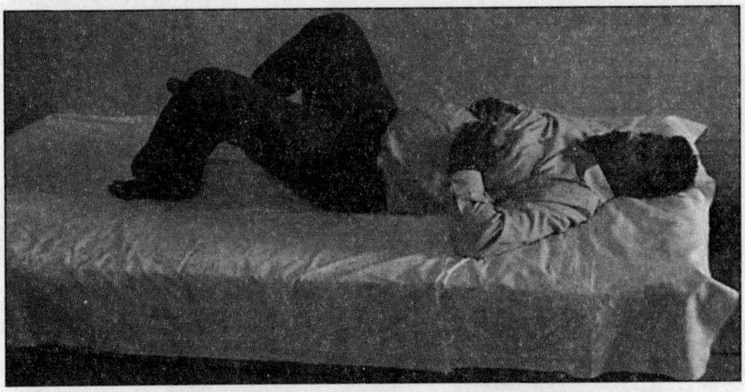

Fig. 18.21: *Tighten stomach and press low back*

Back Strengthening

Begin on hands and knees. Slowly lift one arm and the opposite leg off the floor as shown. (Fig. 18.22) Hold briefly. Repeat with other arm/leg set. Do 10-20 times each side. If this is too easy, you can add weights to the wrists and ankles. Be sure to keep your neck in a neutral position (eyes looking at the floor).

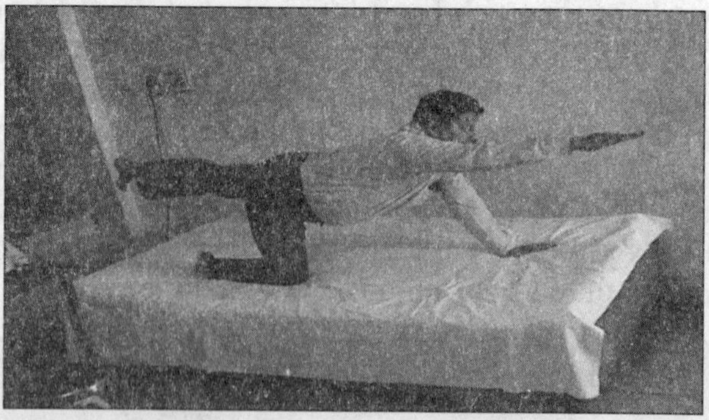

Fig. 18.22: *Back strengthening exercises*

Lunges

This is a very important leg strengthening exercise. It will help make it easier to lift with your legs! Begin in a standing position. Step forward with one foot and move over that leg as shown in figure. (Fig. 18.23) Then step back and repeat with other leg. This will improve your balance and leg strength. It is to be done until one gets fatique.

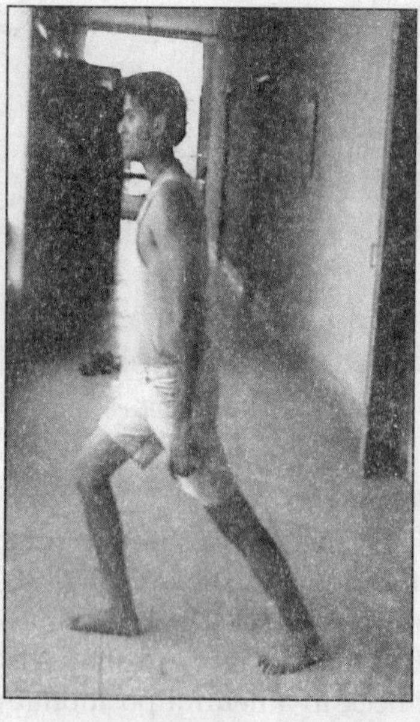

Fig. 18.23: *Lunges*

PNF (PROPRIOCEPTIVE NEUROMUSCULAR FACILITATION)

The basic facilitation procedures provide tools for the therapist to help the patient gain efficient motor function. Their effectiveness does not depend on having the conscious cooperation of the patient. The procedures are used to:

- Increase the patient's ability to move or remain stable.
- Guide the motion by proper grips and appropriate resistance.
- Help the patient achieve coordinated movement through timing.
- Increase the patient's stamina and avoid fatigue.

PROCEDURES FOR FACILITATIONS

1. Resistance

It is used in treatment to increase motor control, to increase strength, facilitate the ability of the muscle to contract, help gain an awareness of motion.

Types of muscle contraction as follows -

Isotonic – The intent of the patient is to produce motion.

a) Concentric – shortening of the agonist produces motion,

b) Eccentric – an outside force gravity or resistance, produces, the motion. The motion is restrained by the controlled lengthening of the agonist.

c) Stabilizing isotonic the intent of the patient is to cause motion. The motion is prevented by an outside force (usually resistance).

Isometric – The intent of both the patient and the therapist is that no motion occurs. This response can be seen as increased facilitation (contraction) or inhibition (relaxation in the synergistic Muscles) and pattern of movement.

2. Reinforcement

The therapist directs the reinforcement of the weaker muscles by the amount of resistance given to the strong muscles. e.g. - the use of resistance in patient treatment include -

- Resisting muscle contractions in a sound limb to produce contraction of the muscles in the immobilized contra lateral limb.
- Resisting hip flexion to cause contraction of the trunk flexor muscles.
- Resisting Supination of the forearm so the external rotators of the shoulder will contract.
- Resisting hip flexion – adduction – external rotation to make the dorsiflexors contract with inversion.

3. Manual Contact

The therapist's grip stimulates the patient's skin receptors and other pressure receptors. The contact should give the patient information about the proper direction of motion. The therapist's hand should be placed to apply the pressure opposite the direction of motion.

4. Body Position and Body Mechanics

The therapist's body should be in line with the desired motion or force. If the therapist cannot keep the proper body position, the hands and arms maintain alignment with the motion. The resistance comes from the therapist's body while the hands and arms stay comparatively relaxed. By using body weight the therapist can give prolonged resistance without getting fatigued.

5. Verbal (commands)

The verbal commands tell the patient what to do and when to do. The therapist must always bear in mind that the command is being given to the patient, not to the body part being treated. The command is divided into three parts –

1. Preparation – readies the patient for action.
2. Action – tell the patient to start the action.
3. Correction – tells the patient how to correct and modify the action.

e.g. – the command for the lower extremity pattern this flexion – adduction – external rotation with knee flexion might be "[preparation] ready, and [action] now pull your leg up and in [correction] keep pulling your toes up" (to correct of lack of dorsiflexion).

6. Vision

Vision helps the patient control and correct his or her position and motion. Moving the eyes will influence both the head and body motion. e.g. – when a patient looks in the direction he wants to move, the head follows the eye motion. The head motion in turn will facilitate larger and stronger motion.

7. Traction and Approximation

Traction is the elongation of the trunk or an extremity. Traction also acts as a stretch stimulus by elongating the muscles.

1. Facilitating motion, especially pulling and antigravity motions
2. Aid in elongation of muscle tissue when using the stretch reflex
3. Resist some part of the motion

Approximation is the compression of the trunk or an extremity. It is used to –

1. Promote stabilization
2. Facilitate weight bearing and the contraction of antigravity muscles.
3. Resist some component of motion.

8. Stretch

The stretch stimulus occurs when a muscle is elongated. e.g. – elongation of the anterior tibial muscle facilitates that muscle and also facilitates the hip flexor – adductor – external rotator muscle group.

9. Timing

Timing is the sequencing of motions. Normal movement requires a smooth sequence of activity and coordinated movement requires precise timing of that sequence. Functional movement requires continued, coordinated motion until the task is accomplished.

10. Patterns

Synergistic mass movements, components of functional normal motion.

TECHNIQUES

The techniques use concentric, eccentric and static muscle contractions combined with properly graded resistance and suitable facilitatory procedures and are combined and adjusted to fit the needs of each patient.

e.g.–Increasing the range of motion and strengthening the muscles in the newly gained range of motion. A relaxation technique such as contract relaxes is used to increase range of motion. This is followed by a facilitory technique such as slow reversals or combination of isotonics to increase the strength and control in the newly gained range of motion.

e.g.–Relieving muscle fatigue during strengthening exercise. After using a strengthening technique such as repeated stretch, the technique of slow reversal is used to relieve fatigue. The stretch reflex permits muscles to work for longer without fatiguing. Alternating contractions of the antagonistic muscles relieve the fatigue that follows repeated exercise of one group of muscles.

1. Rhythmic Initiation

Rhythmic motion done through the desired range, starting with passive motion and progressing to active resisted movement.

Goals

Aid an initiation of motion, improve coordination and sense of motion, normalize the rate of motion, either increasing or decreasing it. Teaching the movement pattern. Help the patient to relax.

Indication

Difficulties in initiating motion. Movement too slow or too fast, uncoordinated or dysrhythmic motion, general tension.

Description

The therapist starts by moving the patient passively through the range of motion using the speed of the verbal command to set the rhythm. The patient is asked to begin working actively in the desired direction. The return motion is done by the therapist. The therapist resists the active movement maintaining the rhythm with the verbal commands.

Examples

Trunk flexion in a sitting position - Move the patient passively into trunk flexion (18.24) and then back to the upright position, when the patient is relaxed and moving easily ask for active assisted motion. (Fig. 18.25) Then begin resisting the motion. (Fig. 18.26)

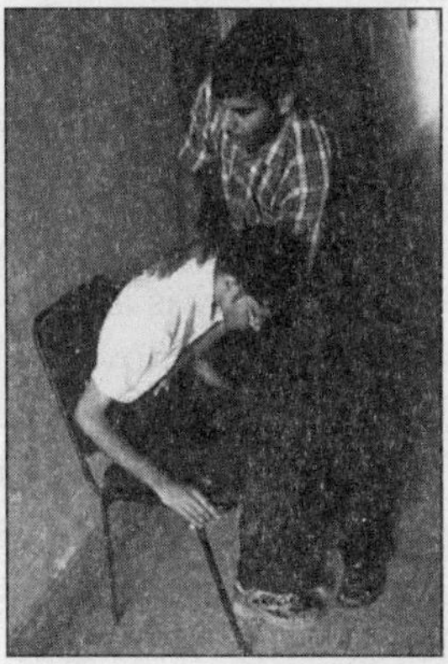

Fig. 18.24: *Passively trunk flexion*

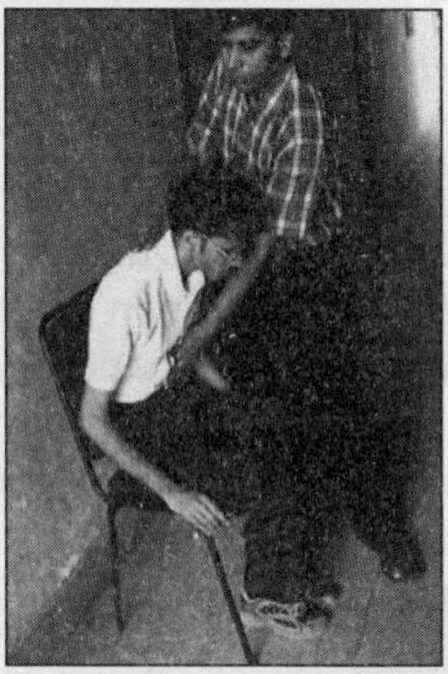

Fig. 18.24: *Active assisted*

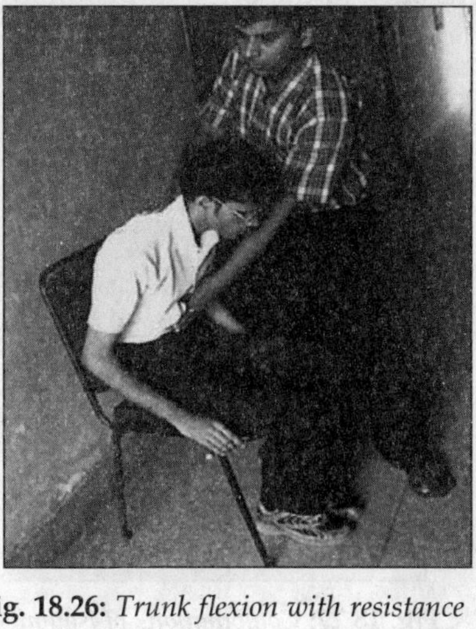

Fig. 18.26: *Trunk flexion with resistance*

2. Combinations of Isotonics

Concentric, Eccentric and stabilizing of one group of muscles without relaxation.

Goals

Active control of motion, Coordination, Increase ROM, Strengthen, Functional training in eccentric control of movement.

Indication

Decreased eccentric control, Lack of coordination, Decreased ROM, Lack of active motion in the middle of range.

Description

The therapist resist the patient's movement actively through a range of motion (Concentric contractions). At the end of the motion the therapist tells the patient to stay in that position (Stabilization contraction). When stability is attained the therapist tells the patient to allow the part to be moved slowly back to the starting position (Eccentric contraction). The eccentric muscle contraction may come before the concentric contraction.

e.g. – Trunk flexion in a sitting position- Resist the patient's concentric contraction into trunk flexion, "Push forward towards me" (Fig. 18.27. At the end of patient's active ROM, tell the patient to stabilize in that position. After the patient is stable, move the patient back to the original position.

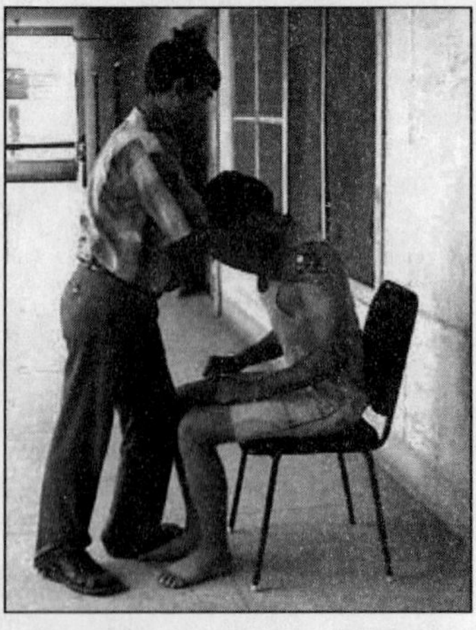

Fig. 18.27: *Combinations of isotonics*

3. Reversal of Antagonists

- ***Dynamic Reversal (Incorporates Slow Reversal)***

Active motion changing from one direction to the opposite without pause or relaxation.

Goals

Increase active range of motion, Increase Strength, Develop coordination (smooth reversal of motion), Prevent or reduce fatigue.

Indication

Weakness of the agonistic muscles, Decreased ability to change direction of motion, Exercised muscles begin to fatigue.

Description

The therapist resists the patient's movement in one direction. As the end of the desired range of motion approaches, the therapist reverses the grip on the distal portion of the moving segment. As the patient reaches the end of his or her active range of motion, the therapist gives the command to reverse direction, without relaxation, and resists the new motion at the distal part. When the patient begins moving in the opposite direction the therapist reverses the proximal grip so now all resistance opposes the new direction. The reversals may be done as often as necessary.

- ***Stabilizing Reversal***

Alternating isotonic contractions opposed by enough resistance to prevent motion.

Goals

Increase stability and balance, Increase muscle strength.

Indications.

Decreased stability, Weakness, Patient unable to contract muscle isometrically.

Description

The therapist gives resistance to the patients in one direction while asking the patients to oppose the force, no motion is allowed. When the patients is fully resisting the force the therapist moves one hand and begins to give resistance in another direction. After the patients responds to the new resistance the therapist moves the other hand to resist the new direction.

- ***Rhythmic Stabilization.***

Alternating isometric contractions against resistance no motion intended.

Goals

Increase active and passive range of motion, Increase strength, Increase stability and balance, Decrease Pain

Indications

Limited range or motion, Pain, Particularly when motion is attempted, weakness in the antagonistic muscle, decreased balance

Contraindication

Cerebellar involvement, Patient unable to follow instruction

Description

The therapist resists an isometric contraction of the agonistic muscle group

- The reversal are repeated as often as needed
- The resistance is increased slowly as the patient builds a matching force

E.g.:

Trunk stability.

4. Repeated Stretch

4a. Repeated Stretch from Beginning of Range

It is elicited from muscles under tension of elongation.

Goals

Facilitate initiation of motion, Increase active ROM, Increase strength, Prevent or reduce fatigue, Guide motion in the desired direction.

Indications

Weakness, Inability to initiate motion due to weakness or rigidity, Fatigue, Decreased awareness of motion.

Contraindication

Joint, Instability, Pain, Unstable 'ones due to fracture.

Description

The therapist gives a preparatory command while elongating fully all the muscles in the pattern. Particular attention is paid to the rotation.

A quick tap is given to lengthen the muscles further and evoke the stretch reflex.

At the same time as the stretch the therapist gives a command to link the patient's voluntary effort to contract the stretched muscles with the reflex response.

The resulting muscle contraction, reflex and voluntary is resisted.

E.g. - Stretch of the pattern of the flexion – abduction – internal rotation.

4b. Repeated Stretch through Range

Stretch reflex elicited from muscles under tension of contraction.

Goals

Increase active ROM, Increase strength, Prevent fatigue, Guide motion in the desired direction.

Indications

Weakness, Fatigue, Decrease awareness of desired motion.

Contraindications

Joint, Instability, Pain, Unstable bones due to fracture, Damage muscle or tendon.

Description

The therapists resist a pattern of motion so all the muscles are contracting and tense

The therapist gives a preparatory command to coordinate the stretch reflex with movement; increased effort by the patient. At the same time the therapist slightly elongates (stretches the muscles by momentarily giving too much resistance. A new and stronger muscles contraction is asked to be resisted. The patient must not relax or reverse direction during the stretch. The patient must be allowed to move before the next stretch reflex is given.

e.g. - Repeated stretch of the lower extremity pattern of flexion – abduction – internal rotation.

5. Contract Relax

Goal

Increase passive range of motion.

Indications

Decreased passive range of motion.

Description

The therapist or patient moves the joint to the end of passive range of motion. Patient performs a strong contraction of restricting muscle for some time (At least 5 seconds), and then relaxation is allowed. This causes gain in range of motion. (Fig. 18.28)

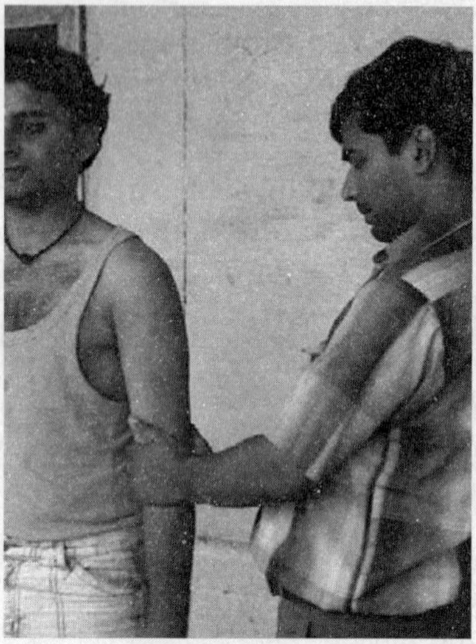

Fig. 18.28: *Contract relax*

6. Hold Relax

Resisted isometric contraction followed by relaxation.

Goals

Increased passive ROM, Decreased pain.

Indication

Decreased passive ROM, The patient's isotonic contractions are too strong for the therapist to control, Pain.

Contraindication

The patient is unable to do isometric contractions.

Description

Isometric contraction of agonist (tight) muscle for 6 seconds and relaxed, during relaxation phase stretch agonist muscle to gain new range of motion.

e.g.: Indirect treatment for decreasing pain in the right shoulder.

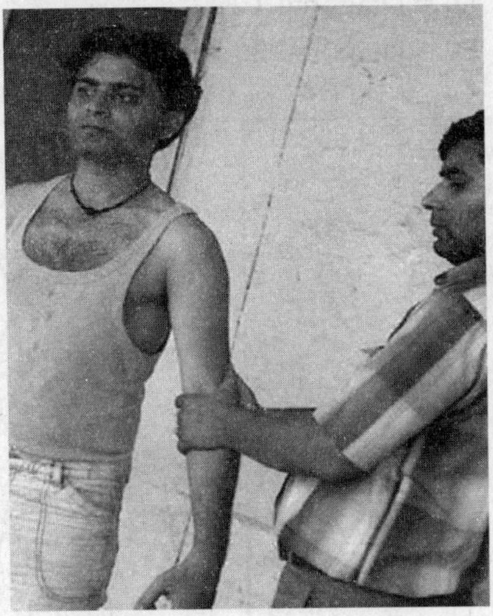

Fig. 18.28: *Hold relax*

PATTERNS

1. **Total patterns.** Also known as developmental postures, they require interaction between proximal components e.g. head, neck, trunk and distal components e.g. Extremities.

2. **Diagonal patterns** used in PNF approach are mass movement patterns observed in most functional activities. e.g.

Unilateral Patterns

a. Upper extremity D1 flexion.
b. Upper extremity D2 flexion.
c. Upper extremity D1 extension.
d. Upper extremity D2 extension.
e. Lower extremity D1 flexion
f. Lower extremity D2 flexion
g. Lower extremity D1 extension.
h. Lower extremity D2 extension.

D_1 = Diagonal 1

D_2 = Diagonal 2

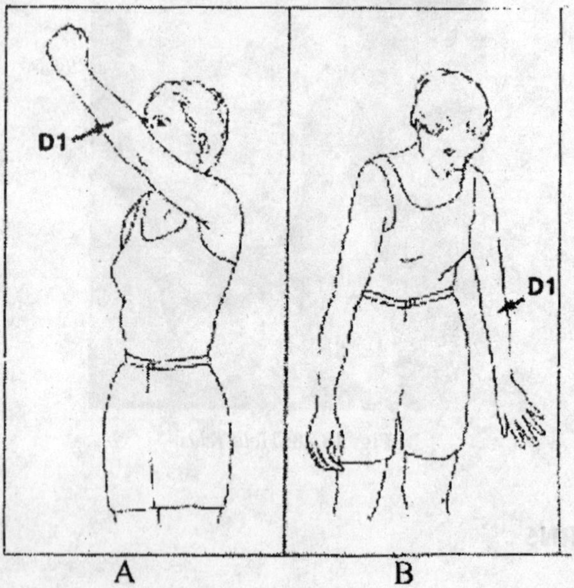

Fig. D_1 : *Diagonal 1 Flexion pattern (A) Diagonal 1 Extension (B)*

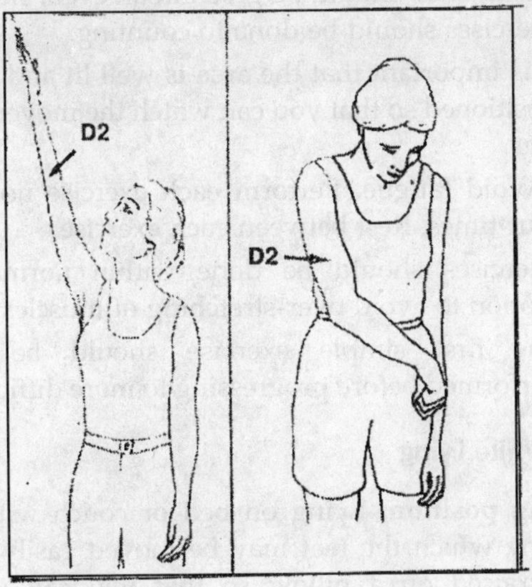

Fig. D_2 : *Diagonal 2 Flexion pattern (A) Diagonal 1 Extension (B)*

Bilateral patterns

1. Symmetric patterns.
2. Asymmetric patterns.
3. Reciprocal patterns.

Combined movements of upper extremity and lower extremity

1. Ipsilateral pattern.
2. Contralateral pattern.
3. Diagonal reciprocal pattern.

FRENKEL'S EXERCISES

This program consists of a planned series of exercises designed to help you compensate for the inability to tell where your arms and legs are in space without looking.

The exercise routine takes about 1/2 hour and should be done 2 times daily.

1. Exercises are designed primarily for coordination; they are not intended for strengthening.

2. Commands should be given in an even, slow voice; the exercises should be done to counting.
3. It is important that the area is well lit and that you are positioned so that you can watch the movement of your legs.
4. Avoid fatigue. Perform each exercise not more than four times. Rest between each exercise.
5. Exercises should be done within normal range of motion to avoid over-stretching of muscles.
6. The first simple exercise should be adequately performed before progressing to more difficult patterns.

Exercises While Lying

Starting position: Lying on bed or couch with a smooth surface along which the feet may be moved easily. Your head should be raised on a pillow so that you can watch every movement.

1. Bend one leg at the hip and knee sliding your heel along the bed. Straighten the hip and knee to return to the starting position. Repeat with the other leg.
2. Bend one leg at the hip and knee as in #1. Then slide your leg out to the side leaving your heel on the bed. Slide your leg back to the center and straighten your hip and knee to return to the starting position. Repeat with the other leg.
3. Bend one leg at the hip and knee with the heel raised from the bed. Straighten your leg to return to the starting position. Repeat with the other leg.
4. Bend and straighten one leg at the hip and knee sliding your heel along the bed stopping at any point of command. Repeat with the other leg.
5. Bend the hip and knee of one leg and place the heel on the opposite knee. Then slide your heel down the shin to the ankle and back up to the knee. Return to starting position and repeat with the other leg.
6. Bend both hips and knees sliding heels on the bed keeping your ankles together. Straighten both legs to return to starting position.

7. Bend one leg at the hip and knee while straightening the other in a bicycling motion.

Exercises While Sitting

Starting position: Sit on a chair with feet flat on the floor.

1. Mark tine, raising just the heel. Then progress to alternately lifting the entire foot and placing the foot firmly on the floor upon a traced foot print.
2. Make two cross marks on the floor with chalk. Alternately glide the foot over the marked cross: forward, backward, left and right.
3. Learn to rise from the chair and sit again to a counted cadence. At one, bend knees and draw feet under the chair; at two, bend trunk forward; at three, rise by straightening the hips and knees and then the trunk. Reverse the process to sit down.

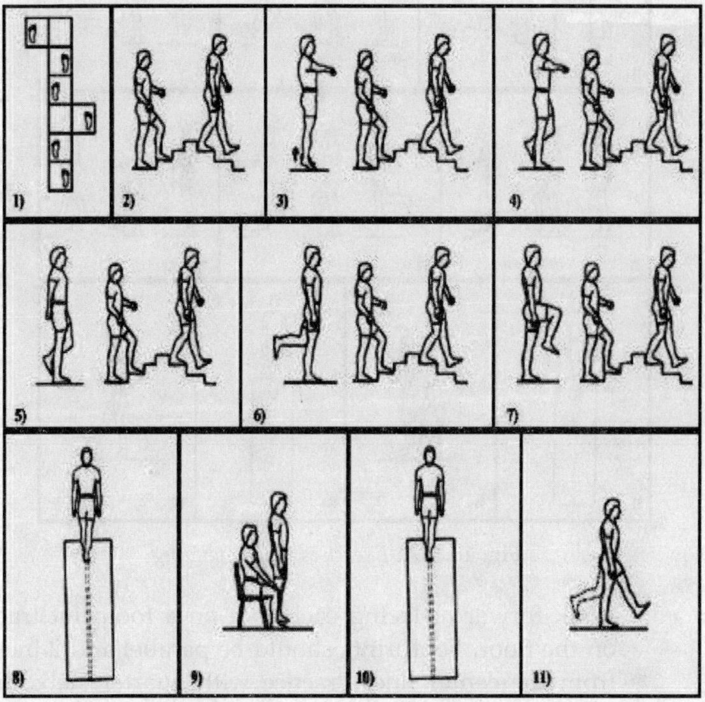

Fig. 18.29: *Exercises while sitting*

Exercises While Standing

Starting position: Stand erect with feet 4 to 6 inches apart.

1. Walk sideways beginning with half steps to the right. Perform this exercise in a counted cadence: At one, shift the weight to the left foot; at two, place the right foot 12 inches to the right; at three, shift the weight to the right foot; at four, bring the left foot over to the right foot. Repeat exercise with half steps to the left. The size of the step taken to right or left may be varied.
2. Walk forward between two parallel lines 14 inches apart placing the right foot just inside the right line and the left foot just inside the left line. Emphasize correct placement. Rest after 10 steps.

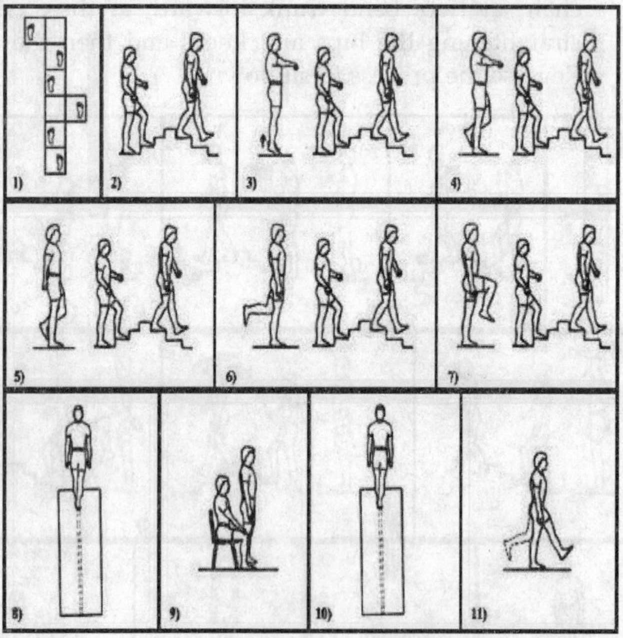

Fig. 18.30A: *Exercises while standing*

3. Walk forward placing each foot on a footprint traced on the floor. Footprints should be parallel and 2 inches from the center line. Practice with quarter steps, half steps, three-quarter steps and full steps.

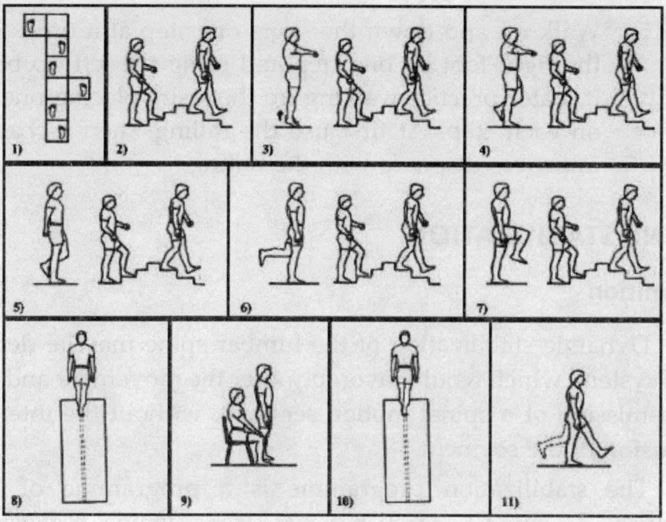

Fig. 18.30B: *Exercises while standing*

4. Turn to the right. At one, raise the right toe and rotate the right foot outward, pivoting on the heel; at two, raise the left heel and pivot the left leg inward on the toes; at three, completing the full turn, and then repeat to the left.

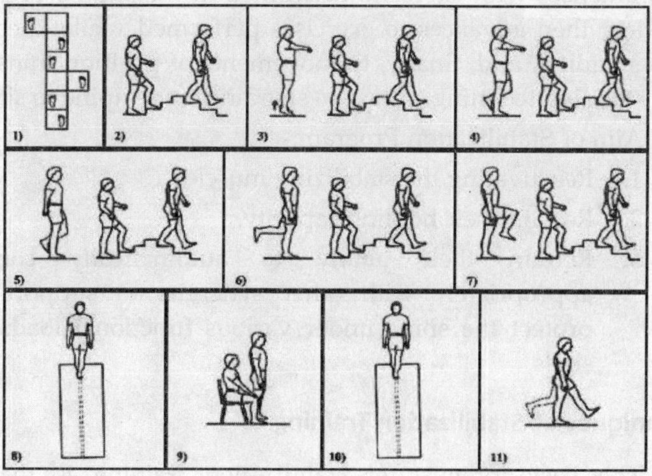

Fig. 18.30C: *Exercises while standing*

5. Walk up and down the stairs one step at a time. Place the right foot on one step and bring the left up beside it. Later practice walking up the stairs placing one foot on each step. At first use the railing, then as balance improves dispense with the railing.

SPINE STABILIZATION

Definition

Dynamic stabilization of the lumbar spine may be defined as a system, which would favorably alter the movement and load transmission of a spinal motion segment, without the intention of fusion of the segment.

The stabilization programme is a programme of back exercises designed to teach patients strengthening & flexibility in a pain free range. Back muscles & abdominal muscles become weaker with chronic back pain and dysfunction may be disproportionate between these muscles.

Stabilization training routines can be divided into basic and advanced programs. The basic program has been occasionally classified as a neurodevelopmental stage of postural control. It commences with exercises performed in the supine or prone position, then advances to exercises performed while kneeling, then standing, and, finally, to movements of position transition (i.e., standing to sitting, sitting to standing, and supine to sitting)

Aim of Stabilization Program:-

1. Reactivating the stabilizing muscles
2. Retrain their holding capacity.
3. Retrain their ability to automatically contract appropriately with other synergist to support and protect the spine under various functional loads and skills.

Techniques of Stabilization Training

The basic premise of stabilization training is that an individual with back pain can be taught to stabilize the painful pathologic condition through muscular development and movement patterns that allow painless return to higher than normal level of functional activities. Because this technique can be used as preventive as well as therapeutic measure.

Tissue Flexibility

- Hamstring musculotendinous unit
- Quadriceps musculotendinous unit
- Iliopsoas musculotendinous unit

Joint Mobility

- Lumbar spine segmental mobility
- Hip ROM

Stabilization Program

- Finding neutral position (standing, sitting, jumping, prone)
- Prone gluteal squeezes with--arm raises alternate arm raises; leg raises; alternate leg raises; arm and leg raises; alternate arm and leg raises
- Supine pelvic bracing
- Bridging progression-basic position; one leg raised with ankle weights; stepping; balancing on gym ball
- Quadruped (with alternating arm and leg movements with ankle and wrist weights)
- Kneeling stabilization (double knee; single knee; lunges with and without weight)
- Wall slide quadriceps strengthening
- Position transition with postural control

Abdominal Program

- Curl-ups
- Diagonal curl-ups
- Diagonal curl-ups on incline board
- Straight leg lowering

Gym Program

- Latissimus pull downs
- Angled leg press
- Lunges
- Hyperextension bench
- General upper-body weight exercises
- Pulley exercises to stress postural control

Aerobic Program

- Progressive walking
- Stationary bicycling
- Running (initially supervised on a treadmill)

The Principles of Dynamic Stabilization

The hypothesis behind dynamic stabilization is that control of abnormal motions and more physiological load transmission would relieve pain, and prevent adjacent segment degeneration. A remote expectation is that, once normal motion and load transmission is achieved, the damaged disc may repair itself, unless of course the degeneration is too advanced.

Stabilization programme can be summarized in 4 stages:-

Stage 1: Isolation and facilitation of target muscles (Multifidus and Transverse Abdominis) Procedure –

- Instruction for isolation and activation of Multifidus and Transverse abdominis.
- Drawing in and hollowing the lower abdomen,
- Drawing the navel up and in towards the spine or feeling the muscles tighten at the waist.
- The visual feedback provided by the pressure sensor provides potent monitoring and feedback system.
- Activation is in four point kneels or prone lying these positions uses the forward drift.

Patient is in prone position the pressure sensor is placed under the abdomen and inflated to a baseline pressure of approximately 70 mmHg. The patients set the lateral abdominals and draw the stomach off the pad, aiming for difference in pressure of at least 10mmHg.

- The abdominal setting action is also taught and practiced in the supported standing and sitting positions as well as supine crook lying position.
- Rotatory resistance applied to the trunk via the pelvis or shoulders will directly activate the supporting muscles with little contribution from rectus abdominis.

Second phase

- Holding capacity of Lateral abdominals & Multifidus. Hold 5 Seconds, rest 5 Seconds, repeating the sequence 10 times and building up the sequence of 10 seconds intervals. Time of hold is measured by using pressure sensor.

Stage 2: Training of trunk stabilization under static conditions of increasing load

Procedure

- Crook lying, low level unilateral legs loads using straight or diagonal lifts. Single leg lift to 90-degree hip flexion and lowering and single leg extension and flexion movement.
- Standing unilateral hip flexion
- Sitting unilateral hip flexion
- Prone lying unilateral hip extension, prone gluteal squeezes, alternate arm and leg raises.
- Self applied rotatory resistance in the bridge position while the patient consciously sets the abdomen.
- Isometric trunk exercises using technique such as rhythmic stabilization in variety of starting position.
- Trunk muscle control in the neutral position of the lumbar spine is trained in a variety of body positions, with four point kneeling and bridging positions.
- Static trunk control in conjunction with other treatment technique: - Lengthening of hamstring in sitting with training for active trunk control.
- Supine pelvic bracing
- Bridging progression – basic position, one leg raised with ankle weights

- Quadruped (with alternate arm and leg movements with ankle and wrist weights)
- Kneeling stabilization (double knee, single knee, Lunges with & without weight)
- Wall slide quadriceps strengthening
- Angled leg press

Stage 3: Development of trunk stabilization during slow controlled movement of the lumbar spine

- The programme is progressed to introduce controlled trunk movement (i.e. movement of the trunk with appropriate activation of the supporting muscles).
- Trunk movement is resisted in each plane of motion. Resistance can be applied to the trunk muscles using body weight and through functional retraining.
  - (a) Curl-ups and curl-ups with rotation
  - (b) Trunk control during back extension exercises can be enhanced by incorporating activation of the lower scapular stabilizer and lateral abdominal muscles.

Stage 4: Lumbar stabilization during high speed and skilled movement

- When the patient's sports or occupation involves high speed or skilled movements, it is necessary to ensure that there is adequate stabilization and muscle control for these activities.
- Progressive walking
- Stationary bicycling
- Running (Initially supervised on treadmill)

Some of the following exercises will be followed for stabilization of lower back.

Repeat : 10 Times

Sets : 2

Hold time : 5 seconds

Session : 2/day

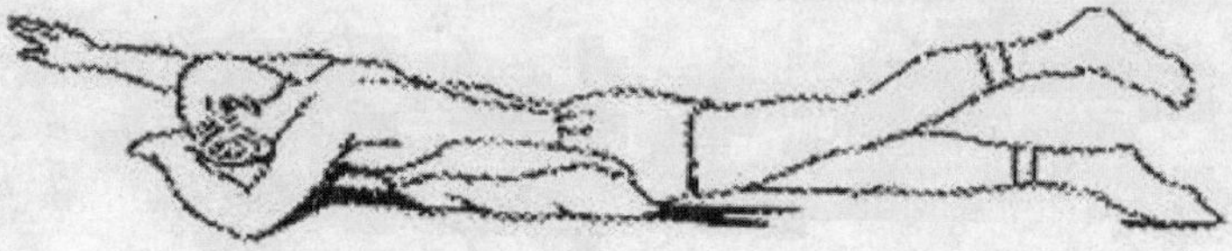

Fig. 18.31 A: *Stabilization exercise of lower back*

Fig. 18.31 A: Patient lying with face downward keep each leg straight and lift the leg 6-8 inches from floor along with opposite arm.

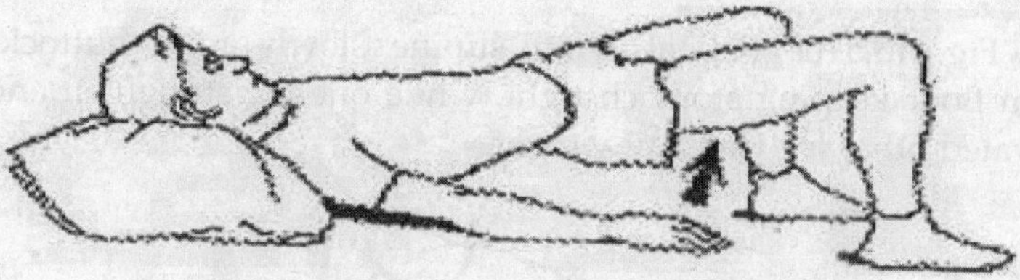

Fig. 18.31 B: *Stabilization exercise of lower back*

Fig. 18.31 B: Patient lying supine slowly raise buttocks and low back 4-5 inches from floor at the same time keeping stomach tight. (Activate core)

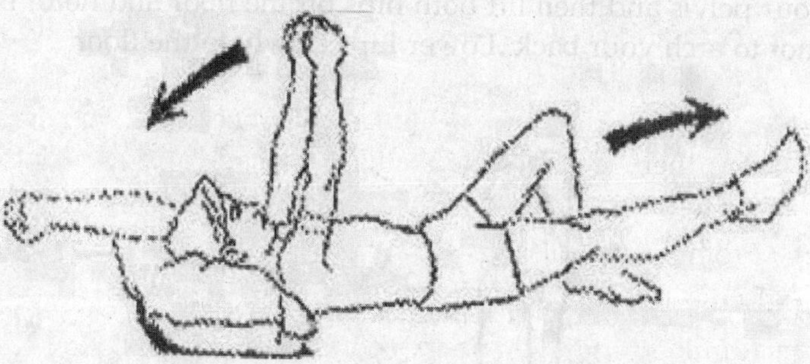

Fig. 18.31 C: *Stabilization exercise of lower back*

Fig. 18.31 C: Patient lying on your back and maintaining a flat back bend both hips and knees to ninety degree slowly straighten one leg out and bring it back to the starting position. Repeat with the other leg.

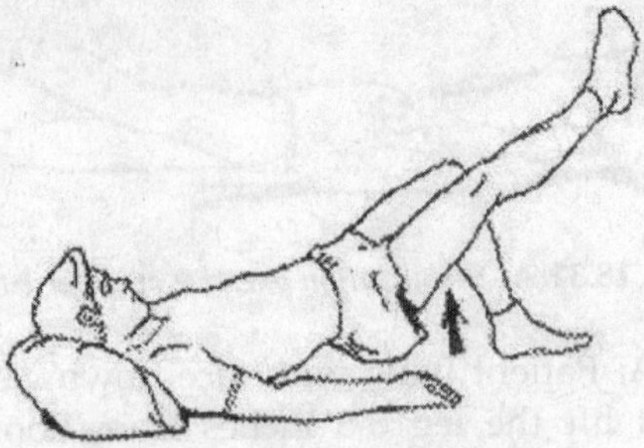

Fig. 18.31 D: *Stabilization exercise of lower back*

Fig. 18.31D: Patient lying supine slowly raise buttocks from floor keeping stomach tight, while one leg straighten and elevated other leg transmit weight.

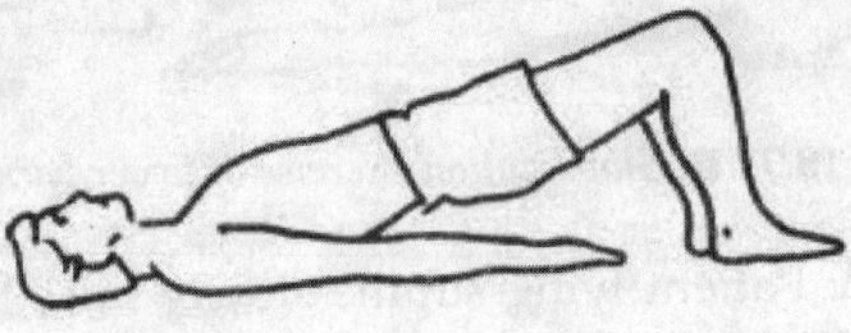

Fig. 18.31 E: *Stabilization exercise of lower back*

Fig. 18.31E: Supine with knees bent and feet flat on the floor. Tilt your pelvis and then lift both hips off the floor and hold. Be sure not to arch your back. Lower hips slowly to the floor.

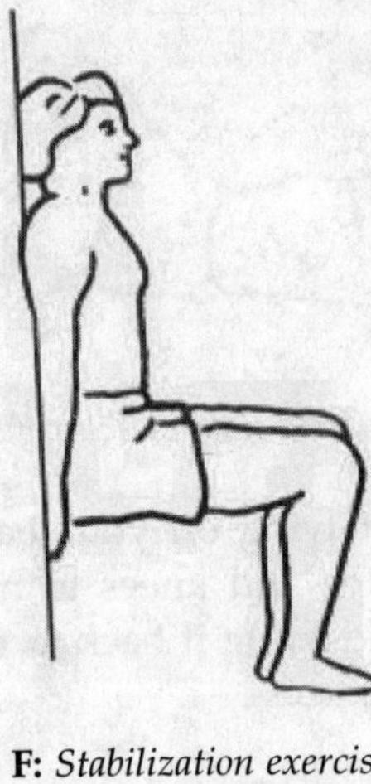

Fig. 18.31 F: *Stabilization exercise of lower back*

Fig. 18.31F: Stand with your back against a wall with your feet about 12 inches from the wall. Flatten your low back against the wall and slide your back down the wall bending your knees to 90 degrees.

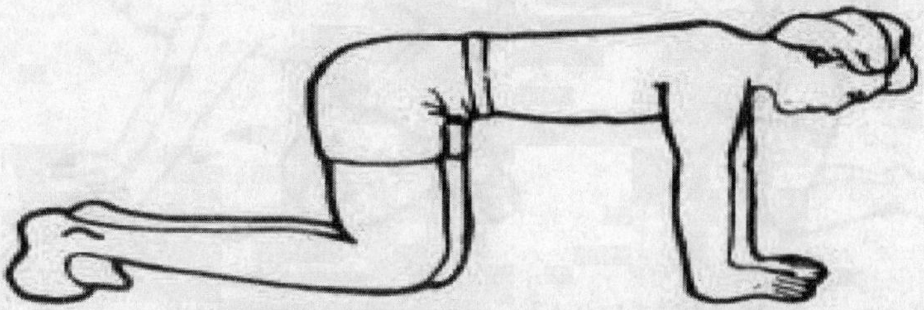

Fig. 18.31 G: *Stabilization exercise of lower back*

Fig. 18.31 G: In quadriped position, find the neutral position of your spine. Imagine you are balancing a glass of water on your back

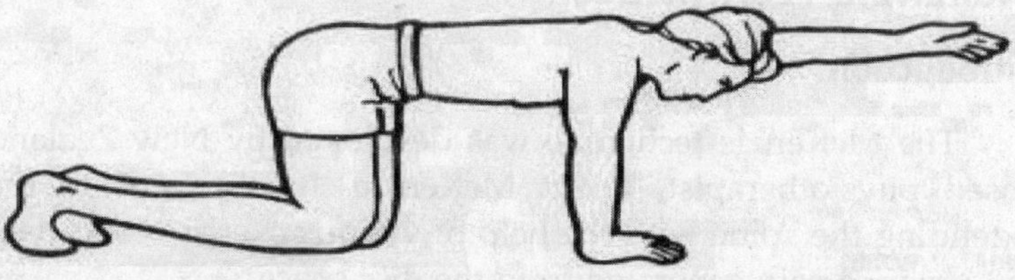

Fig. 18.31 H: *Stabilization exercise of lower back*

Fig. 18.31 H: In quadripad position maintain the neutral position of your spine on hands and knees and lift one arm. Be sure there is no movement in the low back.

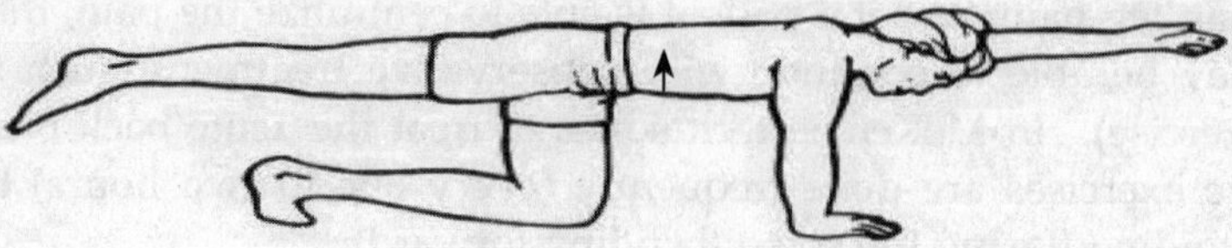

Fig. 18.31 I: *Stabilization exercise of lower back*

Fig. 18.31 I: Maintain the neutral position of back on hands and knees and lift opposite arm and leg.

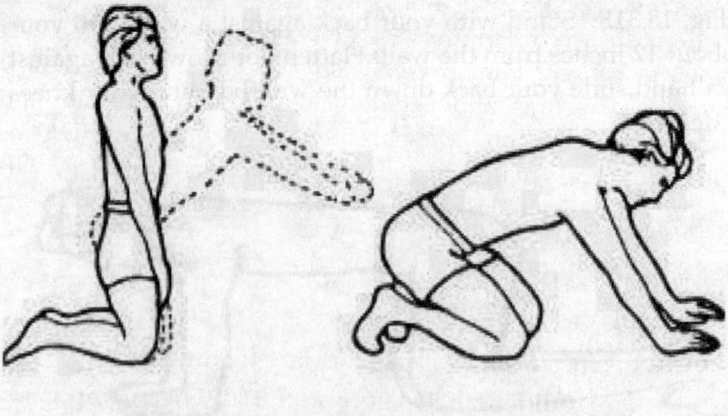

Fig. 18.31 J: *stabilization exercise of lower back*

Fig. 18.31 J: From a kneeling position slowly reach toward the floor. Movement should occur at the hips as you gradually lower yourself to touch the floor.

MCKENZIE TECHNIQUES

Introduction

The McKenzie technique was developed by New Zealand based physiotherapist, Robin McKenzie. It is related to the extending the spine with the help of various exercises and help in to reduce pain generated from the disc space.

In McKenzie techniques, for patients who are suffering from leg pain due to a disc herniation (a radiculopathy), extending the spine with McKenzie back exercises may help reduce the leg pain by "centralizing" the pain (moving the pain from the leg to the back). For most patients, back pain is usually more tolerable than leg pain, and if a patient is able to centralize the pain, they may be able to continue with conservative treatment (such as exercise). In McKenzie techniques to treat the acute back pain, the exercises are done frequently (every one to two hours) by avoiding flexing the spine (bending forward).

Role of Physiotherapy

Patient self-management skills are integral to the McKenzie Method. Physiotherapists teach patients how to perform the specific exercise, positions, and static/dynamic posture corrections shown in the mechanical evaluation to have a direct therapeutic benefit. Patients are also taught to avoid specific movements, postures and activities that clearly increase and worsen their condition. Manual therapy techniques, such as mobilization and manipulation, are introduced if the self-treatment strategies fail to fully resolve the problem.

Benefits of Physiotherapy

The McKenzie method provides:

- Safe, efficacious and cost-effective treatment
- Reliable, differential diagnosis for discogenic and non discogenic pain
- Reliable differential diagnosis for symptomatic and non symptomatic discs
- Self-management skills to encourage and empower patients to use control and resolve their current symptoms and reduce the recurrence and severity of future attacks

Techniques of McKenzie

The procedures include Patient – technique as well as Therapist – technique. The procedures are summarized as below:

1. Lying prone—The Patients adopts the prone lying position with the arms alongside and trunk and the head turned to one side (Fig. 18.32). The prone lying position should be obtained by all patients attending for the treatment of low back pain. It has been suggested that this position can be harmful because it increases and accentuates the lumber lordosis. This applies only in few situations: When we have failed to correct a relevant lateral shift prior to assuming the prone lying position; when extension produces or increases the compression on the sciatic nerve root, and in those rare derangements where nuclear material has accumulated anteriorly or anterolaterally and prone lying increases the derangement. In all other instances the prone lying position is highly beneficial.

2. Lying prone in extension—The Patients, already lying prone, places the elbows under the shoulders and raises the top half of his body so that he comes to lean on elbows and forearms while pelvis and thighs remain on the couch (Fig. 18.33). In this position the lumber lordosis is automatically increased.

3. Extension in lying—The patient, already lying prone, places the hands near the shoulders as for the traditional press-up exercise. This procedure is a further progression of the previous two. Instead of a sustained extension stress on the contents and surrounding structure of the lumber segments, there is now an intermittent extension stress, having a pumping as well as a stretching effect.

4. Extension in lying with belt fixation—The patient's position and the exercise are the same as in third procedure but now a fixating belt is placed at or just below the segments to be extended.

5. Sustained extension—To apply a sustained extension stress to the lumber spine an adjustable couch one end of which may be raised, is a necessary piece of equipment. The procedure is predominantly used in the treatment of derangement.

6. Extension in standing—The patient stands with the feet well apart and places the hands in the small of the back across the belt line (Fig. 18.35). Whenever extension in lying is prevented by circumstances, an extension stress can be given by extension in standing.

7. Extension mobilization—The patient lies prone as for procedure 1. The therapist stands to one side of the patient, crosses the arms and places the heels of the hands on the transverse processes of the appropriate lumbar segment. A gentle pressure is applied symmetrically and immediately released, but the hands must not lose contact. This is repeated rhythmically to the same segment about ten times.

8. Extension manipulation.
9. Rotation mobilization in extension.
10. Rotation manipulation in extension.
11. Sustained rotation/ mobilization in flexion.
12. Rotation manipulation in flexion.
13. Flexion in lying.

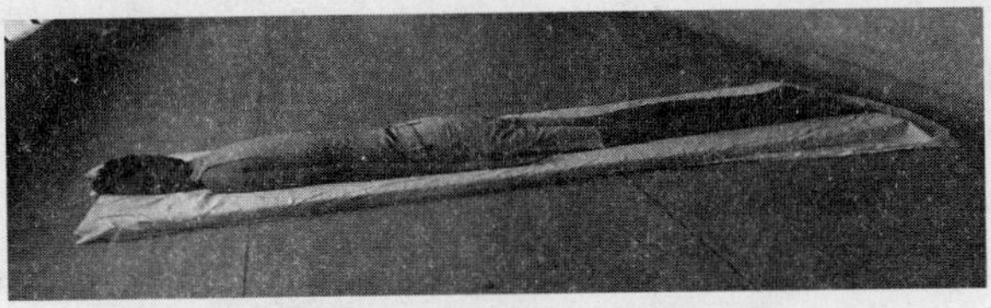

Fig. 18.32: *Lying prone*

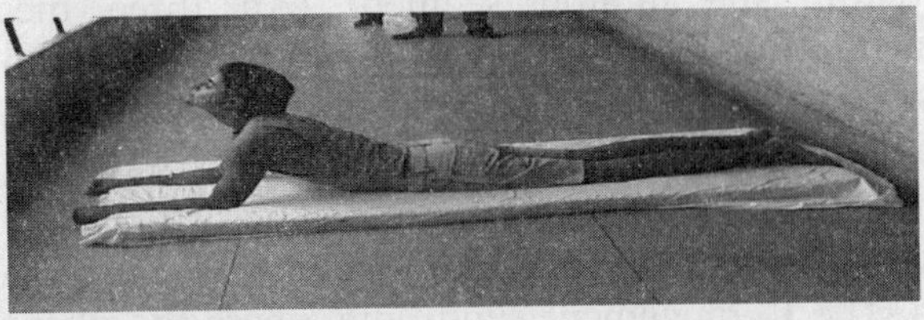

Fig. 18.33: *Lying prone in extension*

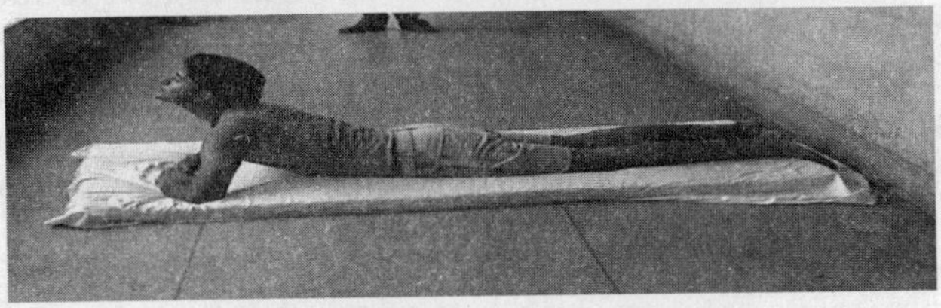

Fig. 18.34: *Extension in lying*

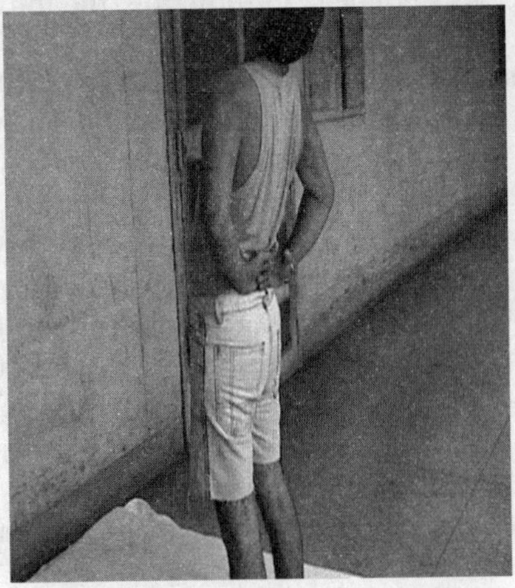

Fig. 18.35: *Extension in standing*

McKenzie described three mechanical syndromes:

1. Postural, 2. Dysfunction and 3. Derangement. (Pain in specific posture)

- Postural: End-range stress of normal structures
- Dysfunction: End-range stress of shortened structures (scarring, fibrosis, nerve root adherence)
- Derangement: Anatomical disruption or displacement within the motion segment (All three mechanical syndromes – postural, dysfunction, and derangement – occur in the cervical as well as thoracic and lumbar regions of the spine.)

Each distinct syndrome is addressed according to it unique nature with mechanical procedures utilizing movement and positions. The Derangement syndrome where the phenomenon of "centralization" occurs is most common.

Well-trained McKenzie practitioners will be able to identify those more difficult cases where advanced McKenzie techniques might benefit the patient versus those patients whose diagnosis is non-mechanical in nature, and those patients are then quickly referred for alternate care, thus avoiding unnecessary periods of inappropriate or expensive management.

Treatment. McKenzie treatment uniquely emphasizes on education and active patient involvement in the management of their treatment in order to decrease pain quickly, and restore function and independence, minimizing the number of visits to the clinic. And if a problem is more complex, self-treatment may not be possible right away. However, a certified McKenzie clinician will know when to provide additional advanced hands-on techniques until the patient can successfully manage the prescribed skills on their own.

Ultimately, most patients can successfully treat themselves when provided with the necessary knowledge and tools. An individualized self-treatment program tailored to the lifestyle of the patient puts the patient in control safely and effectively.

Preventive. Patients gain an experiential education thus learning to self-treat the present problem. The management of these skills and behaviors will minimize the risk of recurrence and allow patients to rapidly manage themselves when symptoms occur.

■

19

DISABILITY AND REHABILITATION

WHAT IS DISABILITY?

It is defined as an existing difficulty in performing one or more activities which in accordance with the subject's age, sex & normative social role are generally accepted as essential basic components of daily living such as self care, social relations and economic activity.

- **Impairment:** Any loss or abnormality of psychological, physiological or anatomical structure or function.
- **Disability:** Any restriction or lack of ability to perform an activity in the manner or within the range considered normal for a human being resulting from impairment.
- **Handicap**: A disadvantage for a given individual in his or her social context resulting from an impairment or disability that limits or prevents the fulfillment of a role that is normal for that individual.

DISABILITY PROCESS

Disability process is the step by step worsening of the health of a person, who is not rehabilitated. It is start with impairment which leads to disabilities then leads to handicaps. If the person is rehabilitated this worsening of health will not happen.

Types of Disability

Two main types:

1. **Primary:** Disabilities that are direct consequences of a disease or condition are called primary disability e.g.

Paraplegia following spinal cord injury, inability to walk after fracture.

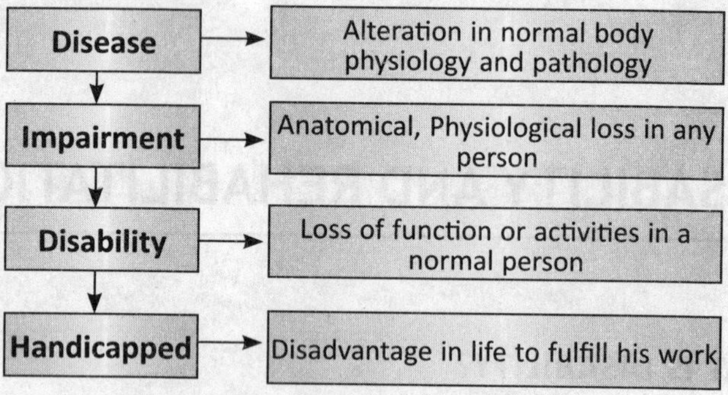

Fig. 19.1: *Disability Process*

Secondary: Disabilities that did not exist at the onset of primary disability but develop subsequently are called secondary disability e.g. joint contractures in poliomyelitis.

Types of Disability

- Locomotor
- Hearing
- Visual
- Hansen's disease
- Low vision
- Chronic mental illness
- Mental retardation

Grades of Disability

- Mild : less than 40%
- Moderate : 40% or above
- Severe : 75% or above
- Profound : 100%

(For all concessions, ability is 40 % or above.)

Disability evaluation is quantification of the residual ability of the individual to carry out his day to day activities.

Causes of Disability

A-Since birth-

- Deformity- CTEV,CDH
- Deficiency - Amelia, phocomelia, hemimelia
- Developmental-Spinabifida
- CP/MR

B-After Birth

- Trauma—Rail-road accidents, Agriculture, Factory, War/ Violence
- Natural disasters like—Earth quakes, Flood etc.
- Infection—Bacteria–TB, Leprosy, Sepsis
- Viral—Polio, GB syndrome
- Vascular—Diabetes, Buerger's disease, Stroke
- Nutritional—Rickets, Osteomalacia, Night blindness
- Rheumatoid
- Tumors
- Osteoporosis
- Postural

Disability Prevention

1. **Primary:** *Aim:* Prevention of occurrence of impairment by - vaccination, proper nutrition, accident prevention, maternal & child health care.
2. **Secondary:** *Aim:* Early detection & proper treatment. Proper first aid, early cataract surgery, early treatment of all birth disorders like: CTEV, CDH, Early treatment of all after birth disorders.
3. **Tertiary:** The tertiary prevention is also known as Rehabilitation which includes physical, psycho social & vocational measures taken to restore the patient back to normal or near normal condition. It involves the following disciplines: Medical, Education, Vocational, Social, and Psychological.

Rehabilitation

Role of rehabilitation is to minimize disability and handicap "to make a disabled person into a differently abled person".

Rehabilitation is combined and coordinated use of medical, social, educational, and vocational measure for training and retraining the individual to the highest level of functional ability. It is a branch of health science which restores function in a disabled person or children.

Medical rehabilitation means restoration of function. Vocational rehabilitation means restoration of the capacity to earn livelihood. Social rehabilitation means restoration of family & social relationship. Psychological rehabilitation means restoration of personal dignity, self – esteem & confidence of the disabled person.

1. Sub acute rehabilitation programmes are designed for children and adolescents who are medically fragile or dependent for care.
2. Acute rehabilitation is characterized by inpatient hospital unit and services like treatment for accidental injury, spina bifida, juvenile rheumatoid arthritis, muscular dystrophy etc.

On going rehabilitation by specialized outpatient services and clinics e.g. services spina bifida, cerebral palsy, down syndrome etc.

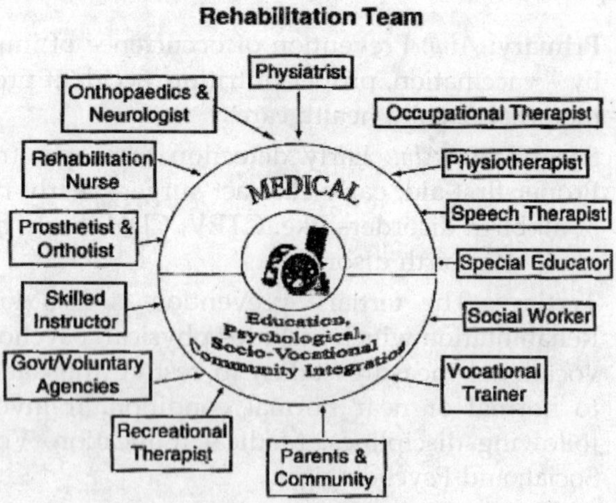

Fig. 19.2: *Rehabilitation team*

20

MAT ACTIVITIES

INTRODUCTION

The mat program involves the patient in activities incorporating both movement and stability. The activities are done in different positions (Rolling, sitting, bridging, kneeling etc), for function and varying the effects of reflexes or gravity. The therapist also chooses positions that can help control abnormal or undesired movements. Mat exercises prefered because they provide large base of support and lower center of gravity.

Exercise mat is a good firmer than most of the commonly using bed, making it an easier surface to learn mat activities.

COMMON MAT EXERCISES

- Hip roll oblique
- Leg Stretch
- Thigh Stretch
- Rolling
- Crawling
- Bridging
- Sitting
- Kneeling

Hip Roll Oblique

Start with supine lying with your hands extended out, palms down. Bend your legs, keeping feet firmly flat on the floor. (Fig. 20.1 A)

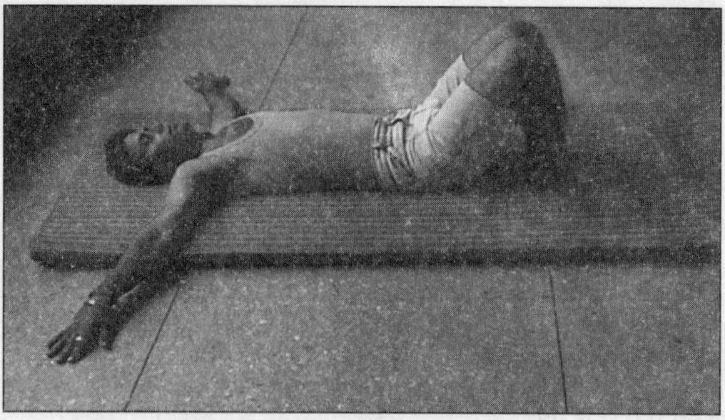

Fig. 20.1A: *Hip roll oblique*

End lower the knees to one side turning at the waist. Aim to allow the thighs to touch the floor, and then slowly repeat again on the other side (Fig. 20.1 B). Avoid lifting the shoulders come up off the floor. Begin by doing two sets of 10 for each side. Increase to two sets of 15 for each side. Advanced aim for two sets of 20 + hip roll oblique.

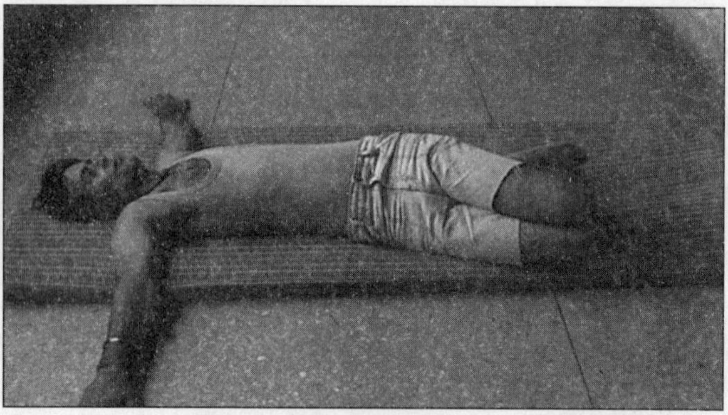

Fig. 20.1B: *Hip roll oblique*

Leg Stretch

Start with lying on mat with one leg extended out in front of you and the other bent in with foot touching thigh of other leg.

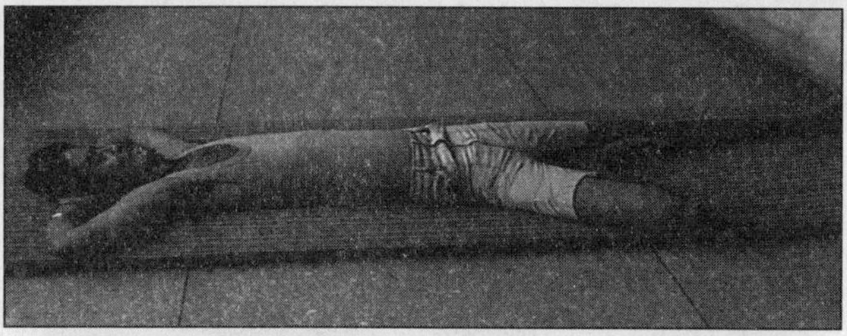

Fig. 20.2A: *Leg stretch*

End by bending your head down slowly away from the extended leg. Stretch your arms down your leg as you bend. Hold for 30 seconds then switch to the other leg. (Fig. 20.2 B)

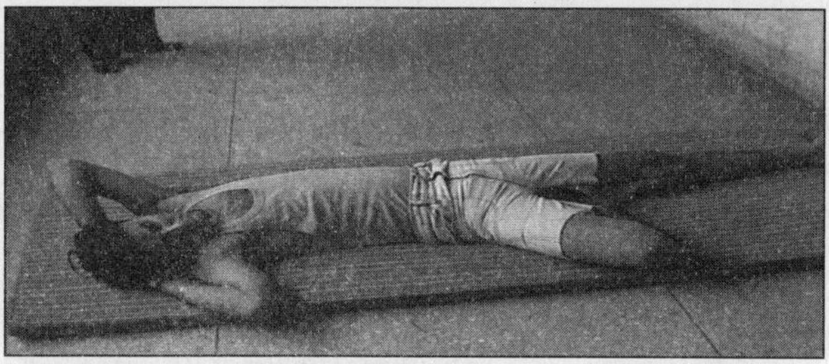

Fig. 20.2B: *Leg stretch*

Thigh Stretch

Start with supine lying; place your right leg across your left knee, keeping your left foot close to your bottom. (Fig. 20.3 A)

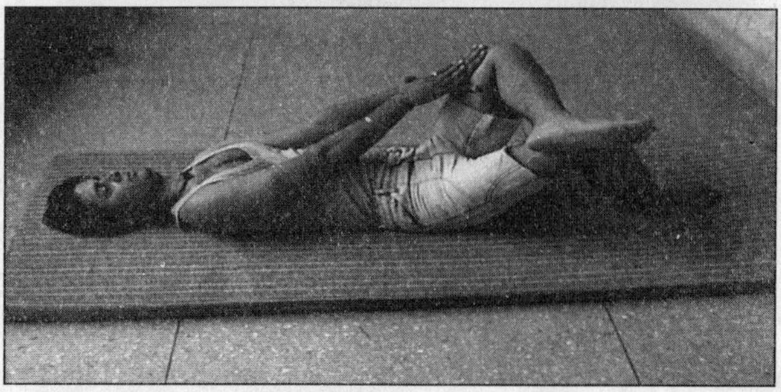

Fig. 20.3A: *Thigh stretch*

End with both hands hold onto you right knee and pull it very gently towards you. Hold for 30 seconds and switch knees. (Fig. 20.3 B)

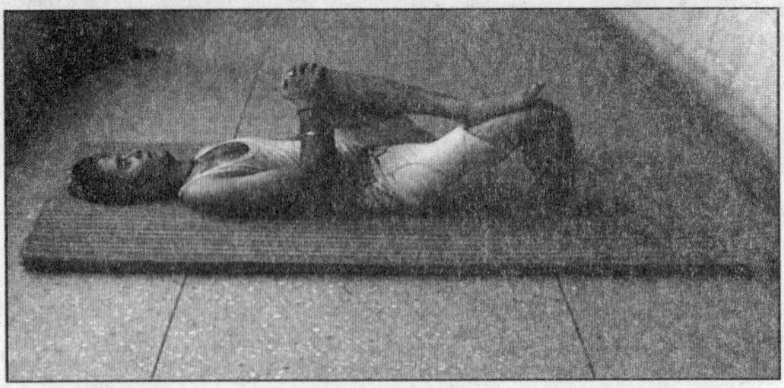

Fig. 20.3B: *Thigh stretch*

Rolling

The goal of rolling can be strengthening of trunk muscles, increasing the patient's ability to roll. Therapist uses either combination of scapula, pelvis or extremity motion best facilitates and reinforce the desired motions.

Scapula

Anterior depression: roll forward with trunk flexion. Facilitate with neck flexion in the direction of the rolling motion. (Fig. 20.4 A)

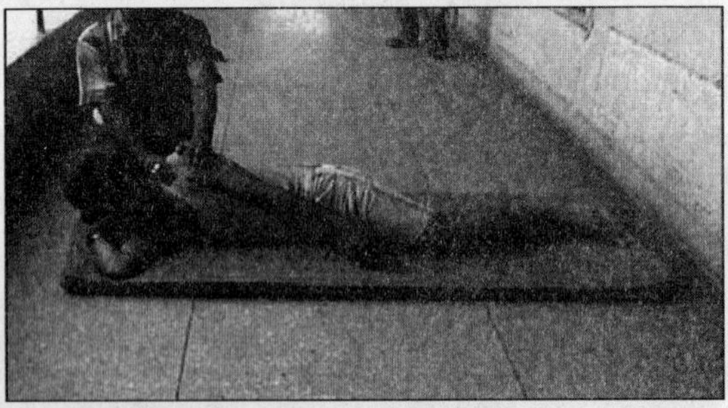

Fig. 20.4A: *Rolling*

Posterior elevation: roll back with trunk extension. Facilitate with neck extension in the direction of the rolling motion. (Fig. 20.4 B)

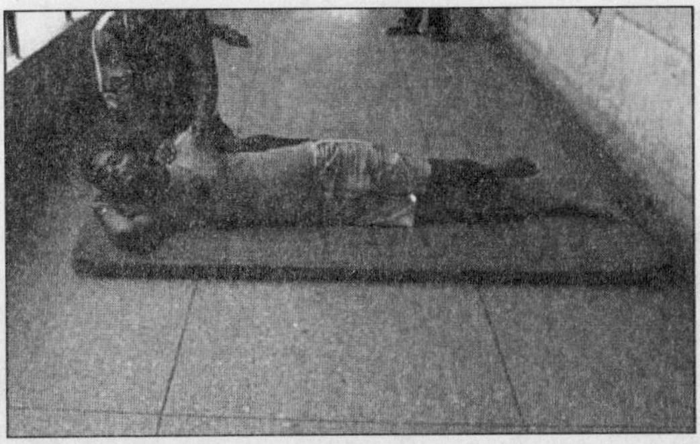

Fig. 20.4B: *Rolling*

Upper Extremity

Adductor (Anterior) patterns facilitate rolling forward, (Fig. 20.5 A) abduction (posterior patterns) facilitate rolling back (Fig. 20.5 B). The patient's head should move with the arm.

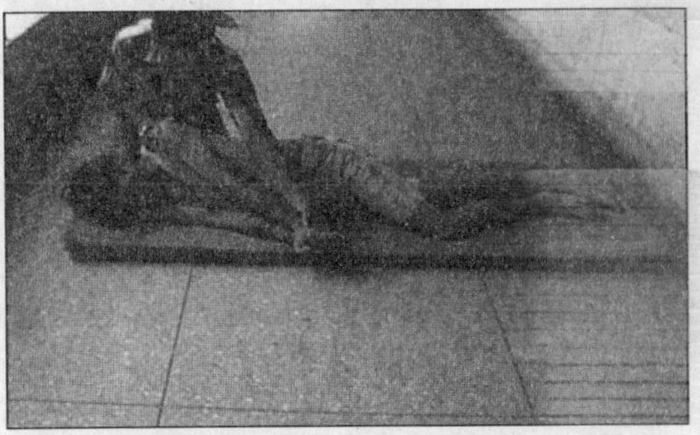

Fig. 20.5A: *Upper extremity*

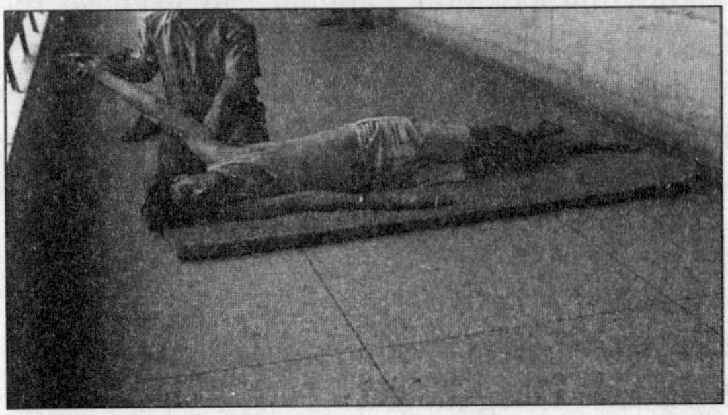

Fig. 20.5B: *Upper extremity*

Lower Extremity

Flexion (anterior) patterns facilitate rolling forward, (Fig. 20.6 A) extension (posterior) pattern facilitate rolling back. (Fig. 20.6 B)

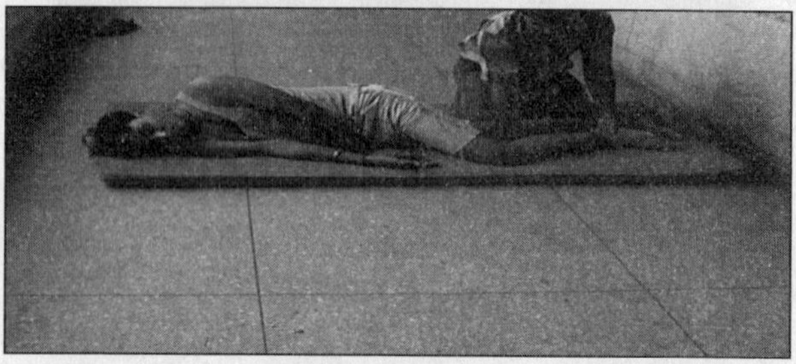

Fig. 20.6A: *Upper extremity*

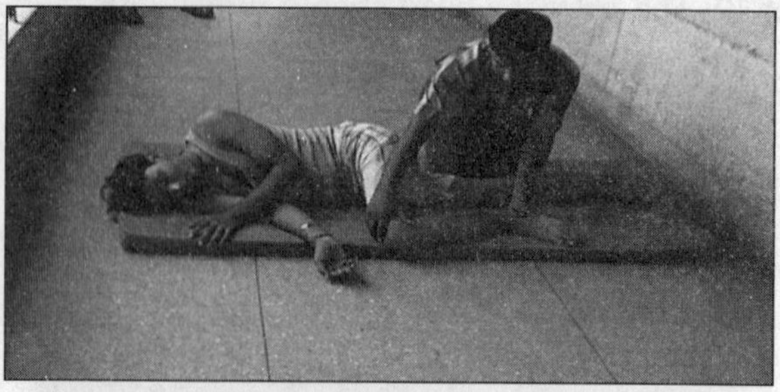

Fig. 20.6B: *Upper extremity*

Crawling

In a crawling position patients can exercise their trunk, hips, knees, and shoulders. Crawling can be achieved with the following exercises:

- Prone on elbow (Fig. 20.7 A)
- Balancing (Fig. 20.7 B)
- Trunk exercises
- Arm and leg exercises (Fig. 20.7 C & Fig. 20.7 D)
- Resistance at scapula or pelvis
- Resistance to leg motion

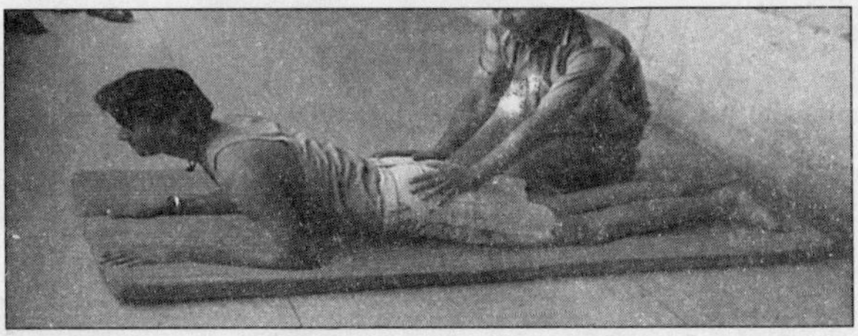

Fig. 20.7A: *Crawling*

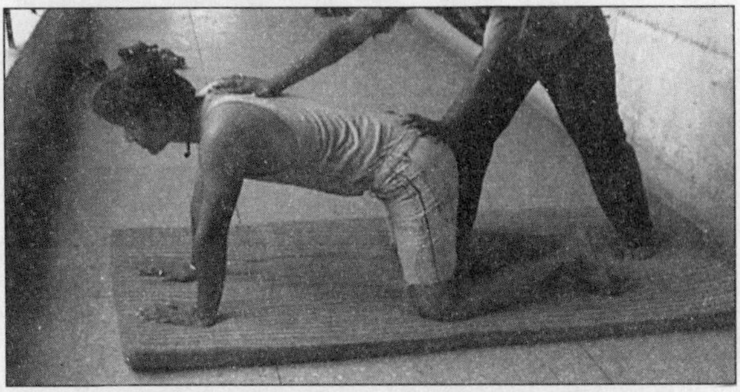

Fig. 20.7B: *Crawling*

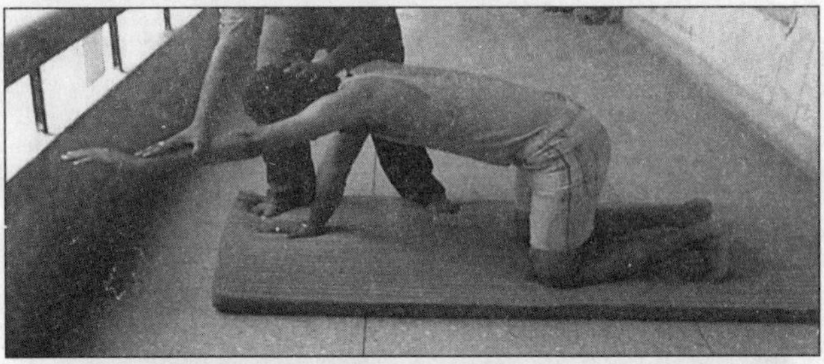

Fig. 20.7C: *Crawling*

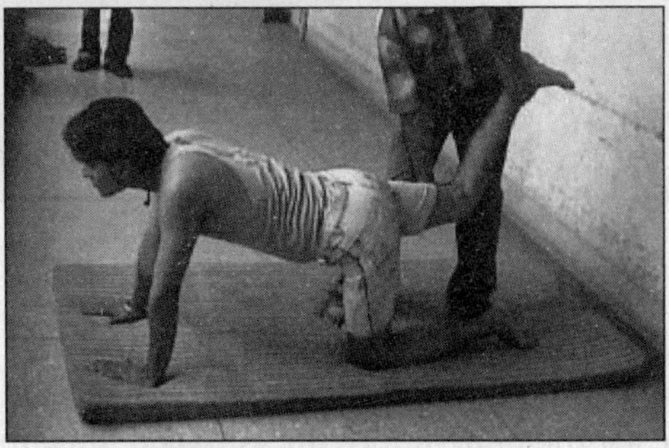

Fig. 20.7D: *Crawling*

Bridging

In hook lying position the patient exercises with weight-bearing through the feet but without danger of falling. Lifting the pelvis from the supporting surface makes it easier for a person to move and dress in bed. (Fig. 20.8)

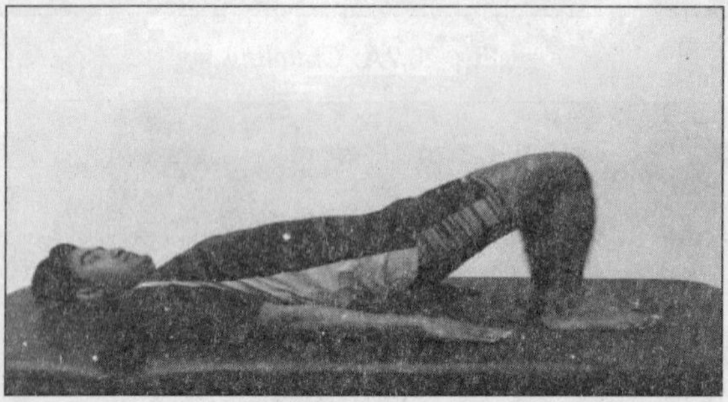

Fig. 20.8: *Bridging*

Sitting

Long sitting is a position functional for bed activities such as eating and dressing. (Fig. 20.9)

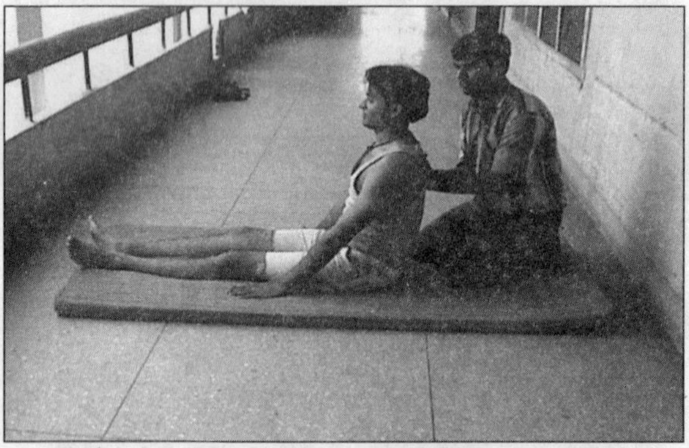

Fig. 20.9: *Sitting*

Kneeling

To increase the strength and range of motion of the hips and knees resist the patient moving between kneeling and a side sitting position. (Fig. 20.10 A & Fig. 20.10 B)

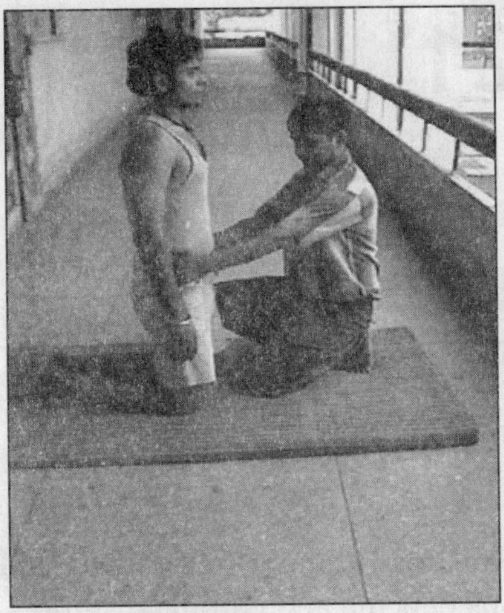

Fig. 20.10A: *Kneeling*

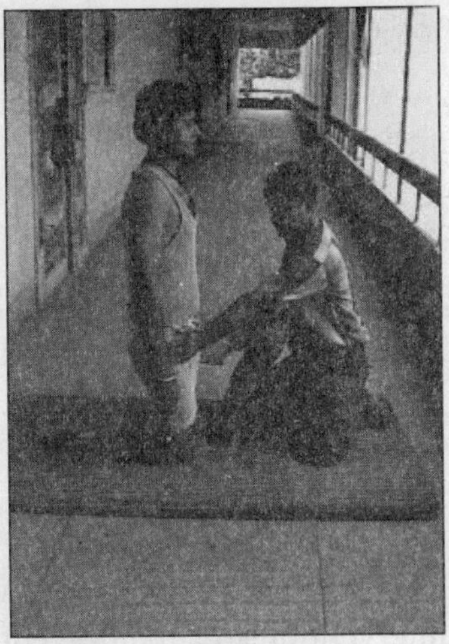

Fig. 20.10B: *Kneeling*

21

BREATHING EXERCISE

INTRODUCTION

Breathing exercise and Ventilatory training are fundamental interventions for the preventions of acute and chronic disorders. Breathing exercise includes following types of exercise

- Diaphragmatic breathing exercise
- Segmental breathing exercise

GOALS OF BREATHING EXERCISE

- To improve ventilation
- To prevent postoperative pulmonary complication
- To improve the strength, endurance, and coordination of the muscles of ventilation.
- To promote relaxation and relieve stress.
- To improve a patient's overall functional capacity for daily living, occupational and recreational activities.

DIAPHRAGMATIC BREATHING

When the diaphragm is functioning effectively in its role as the primary muscle of inspiration, ventilation is efficient. This is helpful in improving efficiency of ventilation, decreasing the effort required for breathing, increase the excursion of the diaphragm, improve gas exchange and oxygenation and mobilizes the lung secretions during postural drainage.

Procedure

Patient is relaxed in a position in which gravity assists the diaphragm as semi fowler's position. This may be coupled with shoulder shrugs to enhance relaxation. Therapist's hands are placed on rectus abdominis just below anterior costal margin. Ask the patient to breath in a slowly and deeply through the nose. Patient should keep the shoulders relaxed and chest quiet and allowing the abdomen to rise. Then tell the patient to slowly let all the air out using controlled expiration (Fig. 21.1 A & Fig. 21.1 B). Patient should practice it 3 or 4 times and then rest. Don't allow the patient to hyperventilate. This exercise should be practiced in supine, sitting, standing positions, as well as during activity.

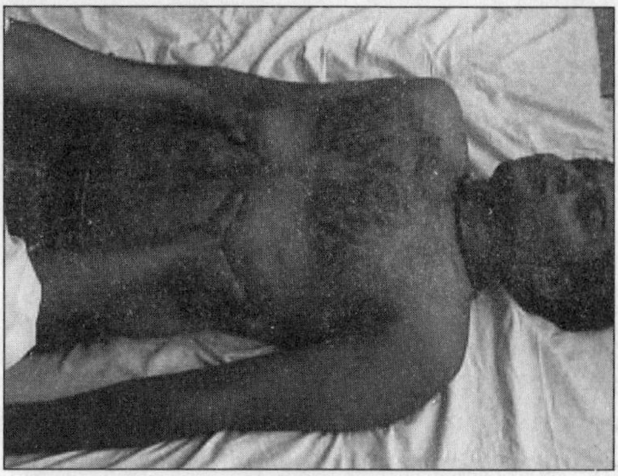

Fig. 21.1A: *Diaphragmatic breathing*

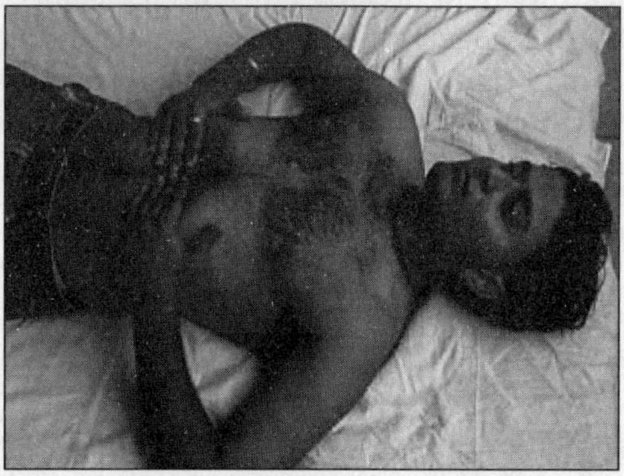

Fig. 21.1B: *Diaphragmatic breathing*

SEGMENTAL BREATHING

When hypoventilation occurs in certain areas of lung because of chest wall fibrosis, pain, muscle guarding after surgery, atelactasis and pneumonia. Then it is important to emphasize on expansion of involved of lung and chest wall. It can done in two ways –

Lateral Costal / Basal Expansion

It may be done unilaterally or bilaterally. It emphasize deep breathing with a focus on movement of this portion of the lower rib cage as it is thought to facilitate diaphragmatic excursion. It is useful for stiff lower rib cage in chronic bronchitis, emphysema, asthma.

Procedure

The patient can sit in a hook lying position. Therapist hand should be placed along the lateral aspect of lower ribs to fix the patient's attention to the area at which movement is to occur. Ask the patient to breathe out and feel the rib cage move downward and inward. As patient breathes out exert pressure onto the ribs with palms. Just prior to inspiration apply a quick downward and inward stretch to the chest on external intercostals to facilitate their contraction. Apply gentle manual resistance to lower ribs to increase sensory awareness as patient breath in deeply this forces chest wall to expands & lower ribs to flare. (Fig. 21.2A)

Then again patient breaths out with assistance from gently squeezing the rib cage in a downward and inward direction. The patient may then be taught to perform the maneuver independently. Patient's hand placed over the ribs or applies resistance using a towel or belt. (Fig. 21.2 B)

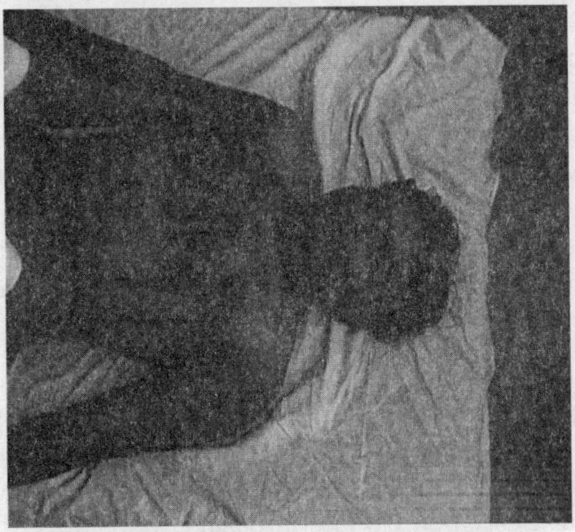

Fig. 21.2A: *Lateral costal / basal expansion*

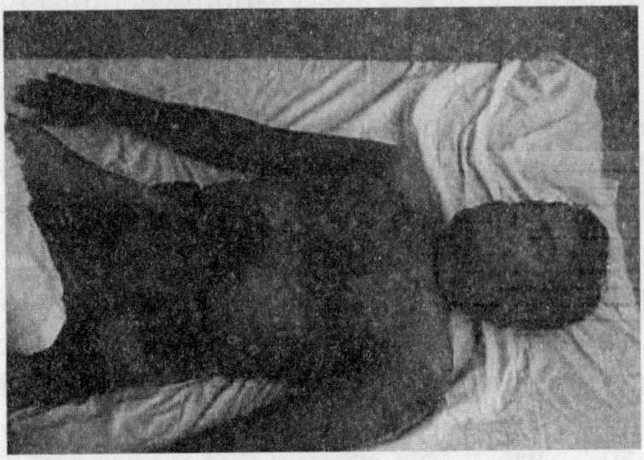

Fig. 21.2B: *Lateral costal / basal expansion*

Posterior Basal Expansion

This is important for postsurgical patient who is confined to bed in a semi reclining position for an extended period of time.

Procedure

Patient sits and leans forward on a pillow, slightly bending the hips. Therapist hand should place over the posterior aspect of lower ribs. Ask the patient to breathe out and feel the rib cage move downward and inward. As patient breathe out apply pressure onto the ribs with palms. Just prior to inspiration apply a quick downward and inward stretch to the chest wall over external intercostals to facilitate their contraction. Apply gentle manual resistance to lower rib to increase sensory awareness as patient breaths in deeply and chest expands and ribs flare. Then again patient breaths out, assisted by gently squeezing the rib cage in a downward and inward direction. The patient may then be taught to perform the maneuver independently. Patient's can apply resistance either by using hands or using a towel or belt.

Right Middle Lobe or Lingual Expansion

When patient is sitting place hands at either the right or left side of patient's chest, just below the axilla. Follow the same procedure as described fro lateral basal expansion.

Procedure

The patient is in hook lying position. Therapist hand should be place along the lateral aspect of lower ribs to fix the patient's attention to the area at which movement is to occur. Ask the patient to breathe out and feel the rib cage move downward and inward. As patient breathe out apply pressure onto the ribs with palms. Just prior to inspiration apply a quick downward and inward stretch to the chest on external intercostals to facilitate their contraction. Apply gentle manual resistance to lower rib to increase sensory awareness as patient breaths in deeply and chest expands and ribs flare. Then again patient breaths out, this is assisted by gently squeezing the rib cage in a downward and inward direction. The patient may then be taught to perform the maneuver independently. Patient' can apply resistance either by using hands or using a towel or belt.

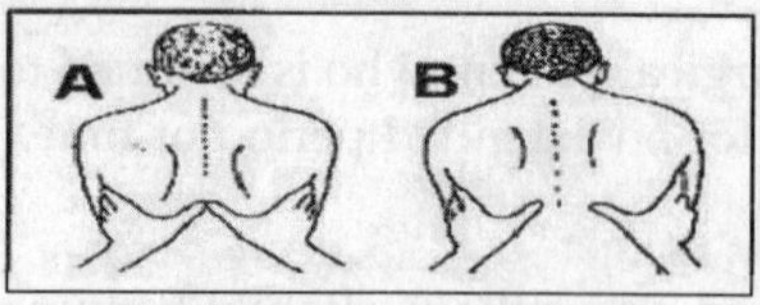

Fig. 21.3: *Posterior Basal Expansion*

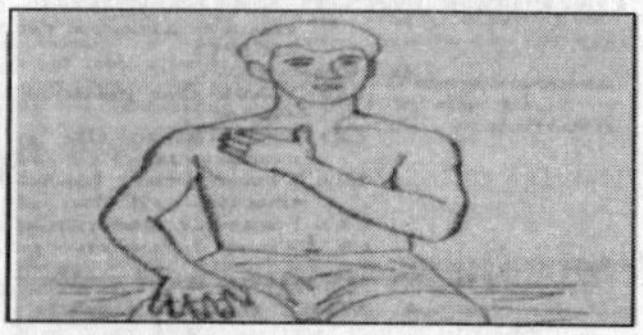

Fig. 21.4: *Apical Expansion*

BIBLIOGRAPHY

Kendall, H.O., and F.P. : Care during the recovery period in paralytic poliomyelitis. U.S. Public Health Bull. No. 242, revised 1939, p. 31.

Lucille Daniels, Marian Williams : Muscle testing – Techniques of manual examination, 1963, p. 1-11.

Roshan Meena and K. N. Arya : Concise Exercise Therapy, 1st edition 2006, p. 14-31.

Porter S., 20015. Dictionary of Physiotherapy, Butterworth Heinemann.

Pandey D.P., Sharma, V.P. Megan Max well 1993, Collins gem, Hindi dictionary, Harper Collins Publishers, India.

Thomson a., Skinner A., Piercy J. 1996, Tidy's Physiotherapy, Twelftjh edition, Varghese Publishing House, Mumbai.

Scottm. Giles M.S., 1999. A Guide to Success, Review for Licencure in Physical Therapy. University of New England, Bideford, Maine.

Griffith, H.W. 1989. Complete Guide to Sports Injuries, First Indian Edition, New Delhi.

Lucille Daniels, Marian Williams, 1956. Muscle Testing, Second Edition, W.B. Saunders Company, London.

Forter a., Palastanga N., 1992. Clayton's Electrotherapy Ninth Edition, Bailliere Tindall, London.

Gardiner M. Denen, 1985. The Principles of Exercise Therapy 4th Edition, CBS Publishers and Distributors, Delhi.

William D. McArdle, Frank I. Katch, Victor L. Katch 200 Essentials of Exercise Physiology 2nd Edition, Lippincott Williams & Wilkins.

David J. Magee 1992. Orthopedic Physical Assessment 2nd edition.

Cynthia C. Norkin, Pamela K. Levangie, 1992. Joint Structure & Function 2nd edition.F.A. Davis Company Philadelphia.

Dorland's 1989. Medical Dictionary 24th Ed. Oxford & IBH Publishing Co. Pvt. Ltd.

Susan B.O. Sullivan, Thomas J. Schmitz, 1998. Physical Rehabilitation: Assessment and Treatment 3rd Ed. Jaypee Brothers Medical Publishers (P) Ltd.

Pathak R.C. 1965. Bhargava's Standard Illustrated Dictionary 12th edition. Shrre Ganga Pustakalya, Varanasi.

Shrinandan Bansal, 2004. Bansal's New Illustrated Medical Dictionary First Ed. A.I.T.B.S. Publishers and Distributors, Delhi.

Michelle H. Cameron, Physical Agents in Rehabilitation from Research to Practice, W.B. Saunders Company.

■